Overcoming Depression
A Five Areas Approach

Chris Williams MB ChB BSc MMedSc

Senior Lecturer and Honorary Consultant Psychiatrist,
Division of Psychiatry,
Department of Psychological Medicine,
University of Glasgow Medical School,
Glasgow, UK

A member of the Hodder Headline Group
LONDON
Co-published in the United States of America by
Oxford University Press Inc., New York

First published in Great Britain in 2001 by
Arnold, a member of the Hodder Headline Group,
338 Euston Road, London NW1 3BH

http://www.arnoldpublishers.com

Co-published in the United States of America by
Oxford University Press Inc.,
198 Madison Avenue, New York, NY 10016
Oxford is a registered trademark of Oxford University Press

Whilst the advice and information in this book are believed to be true and
accurate at the date of going to press, neither the author nor the publisher
can accept any legal responsibility or liability for any errors or omissions that
may be made. In particular (but without limiting the generality of the preceding
disclaimer) every effort has been made to check drug dosages; however, it is
still possible that errors have been missed. Furthermore, dosage schedules are
constantly being revised and new side-effects recognised. For these reasons
the reader is strongly urged to consult the drug companies' printed instructions
before administering any of the drugs recommended in this book.

British Library Cataloguing in Publication Data
A catalogue record for this book is available from the British Library

Library of Congress Cataloging-in-Publication Data
A catalog record for this book is available from the Library of Congress

ISBN 0 340 76383 3

1 2 3 4 5 6 7 8 9 10

Publisher: Georgina Bentliff
Production Editor: Rada Radojicic
Production Controller: Iain McWilliams
Cover Design: Terry Griffiths

Typeset by Phoenix Photosetting, Chatham, Kent
Printed and bound in Malta by Gutenberg Press

What do you think about this book? Or any other Arnold title?
Please send your comments to feedback.arnold@hodder.co.uk

Contents

Foreword
A general practitioner's viewpoint

Most general practitioners need no reminder of the importance of depression, both in terms of the distress caused to their patients and the great impact it has on their workload. In general practice 25 per cent of consultations are concerned primarily with mental health, 90 per cent of which will be managed within primary care itself. Of these disorders depression has been labelled as the 'common cold' of psychiatric problems involving at least one consultation on average in each GP surgery session. Not only is depression an important and life-threatening illness in itself but it is often associated with and complicates chronic physical disease. In addition, depression presenting in the form of physical symptoms may be misdiagnosed.

Improved professional training, together with increased public awareness, will, it is to be hoped, lead to a continuing improvement in the levels of detection and diagnosis of depression, but how will we manage this further potential increase in our workload? Following the introduction of newer antidepressants, pharmacological treatment has become safer, compliance has improved and, it is to be hoped, improving prescribing patterns will have a further impact. The problem of relapse and recurrence of depression, even following a fully adequate course of treatment, remains a serious problem with recurrence rates of up to 50 per cent within 2 years of stopping treatment.

The effectiveness of combining psychological and pharmacological treatment is becoming increasingly well recognised. Of the psychological treatments cognitive behavioural therapy (CBT) has perhaps the best established evidence base for its effectiveness, both in improving the rate of recovery from an acute episode of depression and, more importantly, reducing rates of recurrence by up to 50 per cent. Given the overall costs and commonality of depression there are clear implications for ready access to this effective psychological intervention, but how in practice can this be achieved? Secondary psychiatric services have, for a number of reasons, become increasingly focused upon 'severe and enduring' mental illness. At present there are simply not the resources available in most mental health teams to provide psychological skills, such as CBT, to the large number of patients within primary care who could potentially benefit. Indeed as both a practising GP and a trained cognitive therapist this enormous 'resource gap' is an intense everyday frustration. Furthermore the small number of CBT training programmes in this country, although of excellent quality, can unfortunately still only provide a fraction of the required number of trained therapists.

How then can CBT skills and resources be provided within primary care? Many individual therapists do already work within primary care and efforts have been made to train GPs and other primary care workers in using the more accessible CBT techniques and skills, with some evidence of success. One must hope that this process will continue as the effectiveness of CBT becomes increasingly obvious and these skills become an increasingly important component of the 'primary care culture'.

However, we urgently need more effective interventions now and one of the most promising answers lies in a self-help approach. Self-help books and other materials have a proven benefit in the treatment of depression and the *Overcoming Depression* package takes this approach a further step forward.

Some of the advantages of a self-help approach are the obvious reduction in therapist time and an increase in patient involvement and responsibility. Active involvement by the patient between sessions is an excellent predictor of good outcome in cognitive therapy, whilst the importance of an emphasis on long-term relapse prevention is also well recognised.

Overcoming Depression incorporates all of these factors. There are three additional features of effective psychological therapy that have been recognised. These are:

1 A structured approach;
2 A major focus on current problems rather than past events;
3 An effective therapeutic relationship.

Overcoming Depression provides the first two of these three components and its structure offers the potential for the third. It provides a highly structured framework upon which patients can work through the core elements of cognitive behavioural therapy that have been proven to be effective for the treatment of depression. Its structure is based on sound learning principles with a great emphasis on a thorough learning of the basic principles of CBT such as recognising the links between thoughts, feelings and behaviour before moving on to more involved and sophisticated techniques such as keeping a thought diary. It is the teaching of these basic principles that can so easily be overlooked, even by an experienced therapist. The pacing, reinforcement and repetition are all highly appropriate for patients who may be far from well, with considerable impairment of both concentration and memory. The package also fulfils the second criterion, focusing upon current problems and their interaction with the patient's thoughts, behaviours, moods and physical well-being.

The package consists of manageable workbooks each designed to be read over a one to two week period with the opportunity for a review between each workbook. This review could realistically occur within a standard 10 minute GP or practice nurse consultation. This provides the opportunity for the third component of effective psychotherapy, a collaborative and supportive relationship which may already exist with a trusted doctor or nurse who can motivate and support the patient as they work their way through the programme. This approach gives the package an additional strength well beyond that of simply 'prescribing' a particular self-help book or other material and fits very effectively into the existing framework of general practice.

In summary I believe that *Overcoming Depression* is a potentially very valuable addition to our therapeutic resources and could make a real impact upon the growing problem of managing depression in general practice. I believe that it offers increased hope to our patients and can improve the quality of our own practice and job satisfaction. I am certainly looking forward to using and evaluating it in my own practice.

Dr Steve Williams, MRCP, MRCGP
General Practitioner, The Garth Surgery, Guisborough, Cleveland

Foreword
A nurse's viewpoint

This excellent self-help book brings together an empirically validated psychological treatment for depression with a user friendly written resource. The treatment package uses the principles and practices of cognitive behavioural therapy (CBT) and is presented as a series of structured self-help workbooks that can be used by patients or their health care practitioners.

It is clear from the outset that the author has an extensive clinical experience of CBT interventions for depression. This is evidenced by the cogent treatment rationale presented in the initial workbook and the clinical vignettes that are used to exemplify the central CBT principles and practices presented in the workbooks. The content is informed by the principles of psycho-education and aims to enhance the patient's knowledge and skills in self-treatment. It provides the user with vital information regarding depression, and it provides a readily accessible and easy to follow format. Each workbook provides the user with a step-wise approach to the management of depression.

The overall approach advocated by the package is a pragmatic, problem-solving formula that is the hallmark of this evidence-based treatment approach. The package aims to equip the user with a range of strategies which enables effective mood management, utilising core CBT skills. This includes activity scheduling and graded task assignment, identifying and modifying unhelpful automatic thoughts and basic problem-solving skills. These are presented in a clear, easy to follow format that has been used in primary and secondary health care settings.

The book will be useful to a broad range of health professionals working in a variety of clinical settings. Its most obvious appeal is in primary care where consultation with a GP, CPN, psychologist, health visitor or practice nurse is usually the first point of contact for a client suffering with depression. This highly accessible treatment package would provide a timely and therapeutic addition to the current first line treatment for depression in primary care, antidepressant medication. It also provides an important resource for hospital and community-based psychiatric team workers. Equally the book could be utilised as a waiting list intervention in tertiary psychological therapies services, prior to the commencement of 'formal' treatment. It may prove to be of benefit in reducing the duration of individual therapy contracts, as well as reduce waiting lists.

There is undoubtedly a need for these materials in a day or inpatient hospital setting. In addition the materials would be useful self-help tools in any resource centre, mental health user group or public library.

The book also contains a clinician's guide to optimise the effective implementation of the CBT strategies contained within the package. This follows a similar format to the client's self-help package providing health practitioners with an essential user's guide. It also establishes the overall objectives of the package and equips the clinicians with strategies for assisting clients in maximising opportunities to generalise learning from the book so that they apply it in everyday problem situations.

This book is to be highly recommended as a self-help tool. It is sufficiently flexible to be integrated into a range of health care settings. Its user friendly format makes this a readily accessible package that has potential to increase the cost-effectiveness of services and enhance client satisfaction by increasing accessibility to psychological interventions for depression.

Anne Garland
Clinical Lecturer/Practitioner, University of Glasgow

Foreword
A psychiatrist's viewpoint

There is an increasing trend towards the use of self-help materials. People with psychological problems find self-help a popular format for helping them cope with their difficulties. Professionals are increasingly interested as there is evidence that these approaches can be effective in treating many of the common psychological problems encountered in general practice settings.

Chris Williams is a gifted clinician and trainer who is also an expert in cognitive therapy. Dr Williams has particular expertise in the management of depression and anxiety in primary care and has had an interest in the development of self-help materials for a long time. Dr Williams is in an ideal position to produce an accessible and user-friendly step-by-step guide to understanding and managing depressive symptoms. He guides individuals through recognising their problems, to getting started on resolving problems, identifying the negative thoughts and feelings that tend to maintain depression and ultimately helps them start to plan for a brighter future. The text is readable, informative and engaging. The use of graphics clearly illustrates the points he is trying to make and the use of summary statements, reviews and bullet points constantly helps orientate people even at times when they are finding it hard to concentrate.

As a companion to the step-by-step guide for people who have depression, Dr Williams has also produced some health practitioner notes. These guide the clinician through the detection and treatment of depression and specifically help them look at how to support their patients in using these workbooks.

The combined *Overcoming Depression* client and clinician guides offer an ideal way to start to tackle one of the most common problems experienced by people in the Western world. Dr Williams is to be commended on this self-help package which forms an important addition to the current materials available to people who are depressed.

Professor Jan Scott
Professor of Psychiatry, University of Glasgow and Greater Glasgow NHS

Introduction

Have you ever had the experience of someone you are working with coming back to see you and saying *what you said last time really made a great difference* – yet you can't remember quite what you said? This common experience indicates that providing the right information or question can make a real difference to how the person feels. The concept of using sequences of effective questions and information is the basis of cognitive behaviour therapy (CBT) – which has a proven effectiveness in the treatment of depression. The course *Overcoming Depression*, uses a self-help delivery of CBT. It aims to help the person with depression identify and then change unhelpful and extreme ways of seeing things, and also unhelpful behaviours that might be adding to their problems.

The *Overcoming Depression* course and accompanying section on the assessment and management of depression (found in part 2 of the book) has been written to help health care practitioners offer a structured and effective form of psychosocial intervention within the confines of busy clinical settings. The materials use the popular self-help format, and have been devised to 'do the work' of helping the person find out for themselves the causes and treatments of their own depression.

The workbooks have been devised to act as stand-alone resources that can be used by the person at home between sessions with their health care practitioner.

A note about copyright

The materials once purchased in book form may be copied by the user as many times as required for use clinically or in training.

Acknowledgements

I wish to thank the staff at Malham House Day Hospital, Leeds who have used the various self-help materials over several years, especially Julie Hickson, Mumtaz Ahmad and Julie Tiller. I also wish to thank Frances Cole who has played an invaluable role in co-ordinating feedback on the content of the workbooks within Calderdale and Kirklees Health Authority, who funded the further development of these workbooks, and Anne Garland, Stephen Williams and David Cottrell for their helpful comments. The illustrations in the workbooks have been produced by Keith Chan, kchan75@hotmail.com and are copyright of the University of Leeds Innovations Limited.

Finally, I wish to thank my wife Alison who has supported me during the writing of this book.

Chris Williams
September 2000

Part 1

The *Overcoming Depression* workbooks

Using the *Overcoming Depression* workbooks

The *Overcoming Depression* workbooks have been devised to help practitioners work with people who are experiencing mild to moderate levels of depression, including those who have depression at a level requiring the use of antidepressant medication. They allow ready access to structured and clearly written materials that aim to treat depression. The workbooks act as **stand-alone resources** to be worked through at home in the person's own time and supported by sessions with a health care practitioner. The materials use modern educational techniques and the evidence-based cognitive behaviour therapy (CBT) approach to help bring about helpful change.

Why self-help?

Depression is one of the major mental health problems and is associated with marked personal and social distress. Treatments are mainly either with antidepressant medication or are psychological (the so-called 'talking therapies'). Psychological treatments are popular and have been shown to be effective (Roth and Fonagy, 1996); however access to specialist services is limited. There is a need to develop new ways of accessing these psychological treatments that are effective and time efficient.

Self-help materials are increasingly available and are popular with the general public and health care practitioners. Any good bookshop is likely to have a significantly sized self-help section. Self-help books are often amongst the top ten best-selling books. In America and Great Britain, several self-help materials have been assessed and been shown to be effective. A meta-analysis of 40 self-help studies from 1974 to 1990 identified that some types of problem such as anxiety and depression are more likely to be amenable to change than others (Gould and Clum, 1993). The course *Overcoming Depression* uses this popular self-help format, and also the CBT model which has a proven effectiveness in the treatment of depression.

KEY POINT: what is CBT?

Cognitive behaviour therapy (CBT) is an evidence-based and structured form of psychotherapy that aims to alter the unhelpful thinking (cognitions) and behaviour that is part of depression. The model is fully compatible with the use of medication, and studies of CBT have tended to confirm that CBT used together with antidepressant medication is more effective than either treatment alone, and that the use of CBT leads to a reduction in future relapse. Andrews (1996) provides an overview of the evidence supporting the effectiveness of CBT.

The development of the workbooks

The workbooks have been written by a psychiatrist who has many years experience using a CBT approach and also in evaluating the effective use of self-help materials. During the development phase of the workbooks, each section has been used in clinical practice by a range of health care workers including general practitioners, practice nurses, community and day hospital based psychiatric nurses, clinical psychologists, psychiatrists and behavioural nurse therapists. Feedback from users and representatives of these different professional groups has led to changes and improvements in the workbooks. In addition, text has been re-written to attain a reading age for each workbook of between ages 10 to 14, thus making the materials accessible to most users. The effectiveness and acceptability of these self-help materials are currently being evaluated within a research study, and in addition, training is offered to health care practitioners wishing to use the workbooks to help familiarise them with the content of the materials.

Who are the workbooks for?

The workbooks may be **particularly helpful** for people who:

- are seeing things in extreme and negative ways;

- show reduced activity as a result of depression;

- are not so depressed that they need treatment with antidepressant medication; or

- prefer not to take antidepressant medication.

Please note: The use of the workbooks is completely compatible with the use of antidepressant medication and includes a section explaining the use of antidepressant medication.

In general, the following would **rule out** the use of the workbooks:

- The person is not interested in using the workbooks or self-help approaches.

- Severe/major depression is present with very poor concentration and energy levels that will make reading and the use of written materials difficult.

- Visual or reading difficulties prevent effective use of the materials.

A short section summarising key information on the assessment and management of depression aimed at non-mental health specialists is summarised in part 2.

About the workbooks

One workbook should be completed every 1 to 2 weeks or so. Completing the entire course of workbooks is therefore likely to take between 2 and 3 months in total. At fastest, the person should be encouraged to **not complete the whole course in less than 6 weeks**. Some people will only need or wish to complete a few of the workbooks, in which case the length of time required will be reduced.

- There is a lot of information in each workbook, so the workbooks are divided into clear sections. It is best for the reader to only read one section at a time.
- An important part of the approach is to **stop, think and reflect** on how the questions might be relevant. This is best done by **answering all the questions** that are asked.

- The **sequencing of questions** coupled with the provision of worked examples (using the characters of Paul and Muriel who appear within the workbooks) allows the reader to see how someone else has applied the materials before practising it themselves.
- **Writing down** notes of key points in the margins or in the *My notes* area at the back of each workbook can help the reader remember information that has been helpful. This can help them to **review** their notes during each week to help apply what has been learned.
- Once each workbook has been completed, it is best to **put it on one side** and then **re-read it** again a few days later. It may be that different parts of it become clearer, or seem more relevant on second reading.

The workbooks have been devised to be used either alone or as part of a complete course. The course is made up of ten workbooks. Workbook 1 is designed to help the reader to identify their current problem areas. It contains a simple contents checklist that allows the person and their health care practitioner to jointly agree and identify (though a tick-box) which workbooks should be read or omitted based on their own problem areas and progress through the course. This will help identify which of the workbooks 2–9 they need to read and apply to their own lives. Finally, the reader can summarise what they have learned and plan how to respond to any future feelings of depression by completing workbook 10.

Overcoming Depression: workbook overview

The following table summarises the workbooks contained within the course.

Workbook	Name
Workbook 1	Understanding depression
Workbook 2	Practical problem solving
Workbook 3	Being assertive
Workbook 4	Noticing extreme and unhelpful thinking
Workbook 5	Changing extreme and unhelpful thinking
Workbook 6	Changing altered behaviours: reduced activity
Workbook 7	Changing altered behaviours: unhelpful behaviours
Workbook 8	Overcoming sleep and other problems
Workbook 9	Understanding and using antidepressant medication
Workbook 10	Planning for the future

The structure of the course is summarised in an easily read flow diagram on the next page. You may wish to remove or photocopy this to help plan your use of the materials.

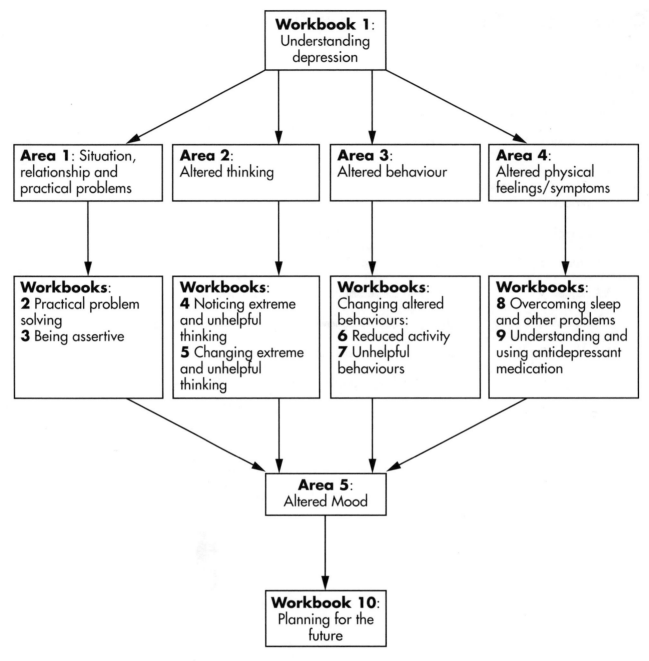

Figure 0.1 *Overcoming Depression*: course overview

Feedback

These workbooks have been created to be clear and helpful for those who use them. Updated and revised versions will be produced based on feedback from those who use the workbooks. Please let us know if you have found the content helpful or unhelpful. In particular, if there are areas within it that you find hard to understand, or seemed poorly written, please let us know and we will try to improve things in future based on the consensus of feedback received. Similarly, if you have found it helpful, please also let us know. We are afraid that we are unable to provide any specific replies or advice on treatment.

To provide feedback, please contact us via:

a) **Our web-site**: at www.calipso.co.uk

b) **Mail**: Dr Chris Williams, c/o University of Leeds Innovations Ltd, 175 Woodhouse Lane, Leeds LS2 3AR.

References and background reading

Andrews, G. (1996) Talk that works: the rise of cognitive behaviour therapy. *British Medical Journal* 313: 1501–2.

Gould, R.A. and Clum, A.A. (1993) Meta-analysis of self-help treatment approaches. *Clinical Psychology Review* 13: 169–186.

Roth, A. and Fonagy, P. (1996) *What works for whom? A critical review of Psychotherapy Research.* The Guilford Press: London.

Workbook 1
Understanding Depression

Dr Chris Williams

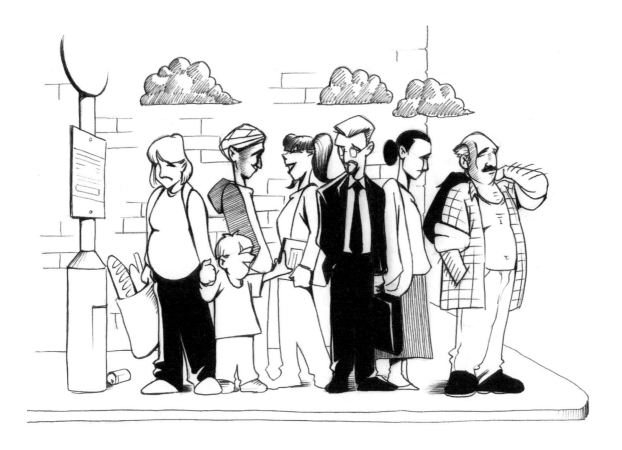

Overcoming Depression
A Five Areas Approach

Section 1 Using the *Overcoming Depression* course

The *Overcoming Depression* course is a series of workbooks that will help you to find out about the causes of depression, and to change problem areas of your life so that you begin to feel better.

Before you start:

Think about how much you know about the causes and treatment of depression. Please answer the following questions:

Q. How good is my knowledge about the causes of depression?
Make a cross on the line below to record how much you know about the causes of depression.

No knowledge _____ Excellent

0   10

Q. How well do I deal with upsetting thoughts or feelings?

Poorly _____ Very well

0   10

Q. How assertive am I?

Not at all _____ Very assertive

0   10

Q. How well do I solve practical problems?

Poorly _____ Very well

0   10

Each of these areas will be a **target area for change** in the workbooks. Each workbook focuses on a different area to guide you in making changes that will help you to feel better.

How to get the most out of this and the other workbooks

This first workbook contains an overview of the treatment approaches people can use to help themselves overcome their problems of depression. By understanding this, you can decide how best to begin to tackle your difficulties.

The workbook will cover:
- how to use the workbook;
- symptoms in depression;
- the five areas of depression: the situations, relationship and practical problems faced by the person, and the altered thinking, emotional and physical feelings and behaviour that occur in depression;
- the impact of depression on you; helping you carry out your own **five areas assessment**;

- the treatment of depression; using your own five areas assessment to target areas for change;
- a description of the workbooks that make up the *Overcoming Depression* course so that you can choose which workbooks will be most helpful for you.

The workbooks are designed to help you to understand depression and to help you to work either by yourself or with your health care practitioner to plan a step-by-step approach to recovery.

The first workbook, *Understanding depression*, will help you to work out which of the five areas of depression you have problems with. Use this workbook in order to work out which of the other workbooks you should read. **This first workbook should normally be read over 1 to 2 weeks.** We recommend that the other workbooks are completed every week or so. Completing the entire course of workbooks is therefore likely to take between 2 and 3 months in total.

- There is a lot of information in each workbook, so the workbooks are divided into clear sections covering each topic. You might find it more helpful to read them one section at a time.
- Try to **answer all the questions** asked. The process of having to **stop, think and reflect** on how the questions might be relevant to you is a crucial part of getting better.
- You will probably find that some aspects of each workbook are more useful to you at the moment than others. **Write down** your own notes of key points in the margins or in the *My notes* area at the back of the workbook to help you remember information that has been helpful. Plan to **review** your notes regularly to help you apply what you have learned.
- Once you have read through an entire workbook once, **put it on one side** and then **re-read it** again a few days later. It may be that different parts of it become clearer, or seem more useful on second reading.
- Within each workbook, important areas are labelled as **key points**. Certain areas that are covered may not be relevant for everyone. Such areas will be clearly identified so that you can choose to skip this optional material if you wish.
- Discuss the workbooks with your health care practitioner so that you can work together on overcoming the problems.

Section 2   **Understanding depression**

1.4

What is a depressive illness?

Feeling fed up and low in mood is a normal part of life. When difficulties or upsetting events occur it is not unusual to feel down and to not enjoy what is happening. Likewise when good things happen, a person may experience pleasure and a sense of achievement. Usually the reasons for low mood are clear (e.g. a **stressful situation,** a **relationship difficulty** such as feeling let down by someone or a **practical problem**) and the drop in mood only lasts for a short period of time.

Occasionally a person's mood may seem to drop for little or no obvious reason and it may be difficult to begin with to know quite why. In some cases depression can worsen and completely dominate the person's life. When someone feels very low for more than **two weeks** and feels like this day after day, week after week, this is called a *depressive illness.*

When depression occurs like this, it affects the person's *mood* and *thinking.* It leads to *altered behaviour* and creates a range of *physical symptoms* in their body.

How common is depression?

Depressive illness is a common experience, which affects about one in 20 people at some time in their lives. You may know friends or relatives who have either felt depressed or have been treated for depression in the past.

Depression can affect **anyone.** Some well-known people have suffered from depression. You may have seen television programmes or read books about their experience of overcoming depression.

What you need to know to understand depression

Links occur between the five areas of depression:
- life situation, relationships, practical problems and difficulties;
- altered thinking;
- altered emotions (also called moods or feelings);
- altered physical feelings/symptoms in the body;
- altered behaviour or activity levels.

KEY POINT

Figure 1.1 shows that **what a person thinks** about a situation or problem may **affect how they feel** physically and emotionally, and also alters **what they do** (behaviour or activity). Each of these five areas (situation, relationship or practical problems, thinking, emotional and physical feelings, and behaviour changes) affects each other.

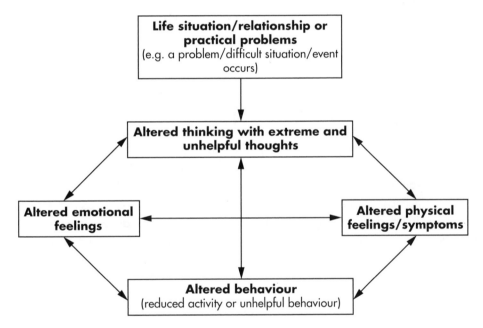

Figure 1.1 The five areas of depression

A **five areas assessment of depression** can help you begin to understand the links between each of these areas in your own life.

Example: How the five key areas affect each other

Imagine you have had a bad day and are feeling fed up. You decide to go shopping:

Situation

As you are walking down a road, someone you know walks by and doesn't say anything to you.

Altered thinking

A number of explanations could be made about what has happened. If you jumped to a very negative conclusion, that, for example, *'They don't like me'*;

Altered emotional feelings

this might lead to altered emotions (feeling down), and

Altered behaviour

altered behaviour (so, for example you might go home and avoid company). In the longer term you might possibly avoid the person or act differently towards them.

Altered physical feelings

You might notice some altered physical symptoms at the time such as feeling low in energy, restless, and afterwards you may be unable to sleep because of worrying about what happened.

Explanation

In this instance, what you **think** might affect how you **feel** emotionally and physically and what you **do**. Yet, there may be numerous other explanations as to why your friend may not have said hello. If you had additional information, for example that they were experiencing problems at home, you might have interpreted their walking by differently. If instead your interpretation was *'maybe they were distracted or upset and just didn't see me'* (altered thinking) and you believed this 100 per cent, it's likely that you might feel very differently about what happened. You might be more likely to feel sorry (altered feelings) for the person. You probably wouldn't experience as many or as strong physical symptoms (altered physical symptoms) and it is also unlikely that you would avoid seeing them again (altered behaviour). In fact, it's possible you might go out of your way to contact them.

In this example, what you **think** affects how you **feel** and what you **do**.

KEY POINT

This example shows that it is not events themselves that cause depression, but the **interpretation** that people make of the event. In depression, the person has more extreme, negative and unhelpful thinking styles. These thoughts build up out of all proportion, and affect how the person feels and what they do.

Q. How helpful is this model in understanding how you feel?

Not at all _____ Extremely helpful

0   10

You will now have a chance to look at how depression is affecting you in each of these five areas by carrying out your own five areas assessment.

Symptoms in depression: the five areas assessment

A **five areas assessment** can be helpful in beginning to understand your symptoms of depression, and in choosing targets for change:

- situation, relationship or practical problems;
- altered thinking;
- altered behaviour (reduced activity or unhelpful behaviours);
- altered physical symptoms;
- altered mood.

You will now have the opportunity to find out more about each of the five areas.

KEY POINT

As you go through the following questions, try hard to really think about your answers. Don't rush though the questions, instead, try to **answer all the questions** so that you are really thinking about how what you read might apply to you.

Area 1: Situation, relationship and practical problems contributing to depression

All of us from time to time face practical problems and difficulties. The actions of important people around us can also create upsets and difficulties. Practical problems such as relationship or financial difficulties may also be present. When someone faces a large number of problems they may begin to feel overwhelmed and depressed. Dwelling on the problems may worsen things still further and quickly get them out of all proportion. The problem is unhelpfully focused on and mulled over again and again in a way that doesn't help resolve it.

An **unhelpful focus** can worsen how you feel and leave you unable to know where to start to change things.

Practical problems may include:

- debts, housing or other difficulties;

- problems in relationships with family, friends or colleagues etc;

- other difficult situations that you face.

Part of the assessment is to consider how these different factors may be affecting you.

Feelings of depression are often linked to **stresses** at home or work (or lack of work – for example **unemployment**). People who have suffered a relationship split, or who feel isolated with no one to talk to about how they feel are also prone to depression. Young mothers, and mothers facing the demands of trying to bring up many young children are also at greater risk of depression. At the same time, practical and helpful supports may be available through friends or relatives.

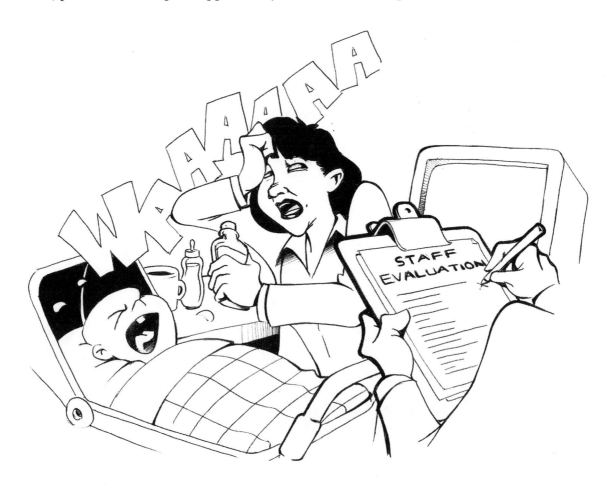

The following table summarises several common factors that may be associated with depression. Are any of these relevant to you?

Situation, relationship and practical problems

I have relationship difficulties (such as arguments) with:	Yes ☐	No ☐

✎ *(Write in the person's name or initials)*

I can't really talk and receive support from my partner.	Yes ☐	No ☐
There is no one around who I can really talk to.	Yes ☐	No ☐
I feel stressed by the demands of looking after my children.	Yes ☐	No ☐
I have difficulties with money worries or debts.	Yes ☐	No ☐
I don't like where I live.	Yes ☐	No ☐
I am having problems with my neighbours.	Yes ☐	No ☐
I feel upset by my lack of a job.	Yes ☐	No ☐
I don't enjoy my job.	Yes ☐	No ☐
I have difficulties with colleagues at work.	Yes ☐	No ☐

Summary for Area 1

Having answered these questions:

Q. Overall, do I have problems in this area?   Yes ☐   No ☐

Area 2: Altered thinking in depression
Unhelpful thinking styles
In depression, it can seem that everything is viewed in a negative way. This might include:

a) A bias against yourself

The person is very negative and is full of self-blame and critical self-talk. Nothing they do is right. They are their own worst critic.
(E.g. 'I'm useless', 'I mess everything up'.)

b) Putting a negative slant on things

Overlooking or downplaying the positive and focusing instead on the negative side of every situation commonly occurs in depression. It is as if the person has a mental filter that focuses only on the negative – a **negative mental filter.**
(E.g. 'The last week was completely awful. Nothing went right'.)

c) Having a gloomy view of the future

Making **negative predictions** about the future or worrying that the worst will happen. This may include a loss of hope, or suicidal ideas.
(E.g. 'I'm not going to visit my friends – I wouldn't enjoy it'.)

Sometimes, this process of predicting that the very worst will happen is called **catastrophic thinking**. This can worsen how you feel and unhelpfully alter what you do.

d) Negative view about how others see you

Second-guessing or mind-reading that others don't like you or see you as weak, stupid or useless. Usually, the person does not actually try to find out if their fears are true.
(E.g. 'She thinks I'm an idiot'.)

e) Bearing all responsibility

Unfairly taking responsibility for things. The person feels the pressure for things to go well, and blames themselves if things don't go as expected **even if** they are not really to blame.
(E.g. 'I'll ruin the evening for everybody and it will be all my fault'.)

f) Making extreme statements or rules

Very strong statements are made, e.g. *'It was* **completely** *useless'* even when what actually happened wasn't anywhere near that bad. The person may also set themselves impossible targets which no one could possibly meet *(e.g. 'It must be* **completely** *perfect, anything less will mean* **total** *failure')*. This thinking style causes the person to use the words *should, got to, must* and *ought* a lot, and also very strong statements such as *always, never* (e.g. *'I never do things well'*) and *typical* (e.g. *'just typical, everything always goes wrong'*).

KEY POINT

These unhelpful thinking styles are important because they tend to reflect consistent **unhelpful thinking styles** that you do again and again. Beginning to notice these and challenge them is an important part of change. All these styles tend to be:

- extreme, with **black or white** thinking.
- **unhelpful,** with a focus on negative things and events that can worsen how you feel.

My thinking style

Think about whether you notice these thinking styles in your own life:

> **Q. Do I have negative or extreme thoughts at times?**
>
> Please answer the following questions and **tick yes** if you have found yourself having negative thoughts like these in the last week.

a) Am I biased against myself?

Have you have noticed any times during the last week when you have been biased against yourself? You may have focused on the negative in things or seen everything through dark tinted glasses.

Q. Am I my own worst critic?   Yes ☐   No ☐

Q. Do I focus on my weaknesses?   Yes ☐   No ☐

Q. Do you recognise any of the following self-statements?

I messed that up   Yes ☐   No ☐

I'm stupid   Yes ☐   No ☐

I can't do anything right   Yes ☐   No ☐

Q. Have you noticed any other kinds of bias against yourself?

✎ Write here the example(s) you noticed:

---

b) Putting a negative slant on things – negative mental filter

Have you have noticed any times during the last week when you have put a negative slant on things?

Q. Do I tend to focus on the bad in situations?   Yes ☐   No ☐

Q. Do I downplay my achievements?   Yes ☐   No ☐

Q. Do you recognise any of the following thoughts?

That was a complete waste of time   Yes ☐   No ☐

The entire week has gone badly   Yes ☐   No ☐

Nothing ever goes right   Yes ☐   No ☐

This process of putting a negative 'spin' on everything is called a negative mental filter.

Q. Have you noticed any other examples of the negative mental filter?

✎ Write here the example(s) you noticed:

c) Having a gloomy view of the future – making negative predictions

Have you have noticed any times during the last week when you have made negative predictions about how things will turn out?

Q. Do I make negative predictions about the future? Yes ☐ No ☐

Q. Do I predict that things will go wrong? Yes ☐ No☐

Q. Do I ever feel hopeless as if things can't get better? Yes ☐ No ☐

Q. Do I ever feel suicidal? Yes ☐ No ☐

Q. Have you noticed any of the following negative predictions in the last week?

I won't enjoy it so what's the point? Yes ☐ No ☐

Nothing will make any difference Yes ☐ No ☐

It will be a complete disaster Yes ☐ No ☐

Q. Have you noticed any other examples of making negative predictions or catastrophic thinking?

✎ Write here any example(s) you noticed:

```
[                                              ]
```

d) Negative view about how others see me – do I mind-read?

Q. Do you second-guess or mind-read that others think badly of you?

Q. Do I second guess or *mind-read* what others think of me? Yes ☐ No ☐

Q. Do I often think that others don't like me? Yes ☐ No ☐

Q. Do you recognise any of the following examples of mind-reading in the last week?

Nobody cares Yes ☐ No ☐

Nobody likes me Yes ☐ No ☐

He/she/they think badly of me Yes ☐ No ☐

Mind-reading can worsen how you **feel** and unhelpfully alter what you **do**.

Q. Have you noticed other examples of mind-reading?

✎ Write here the example(s) you noticed:

```
[                                              ]
```

e) Bearing all responsibility

Q. Have you felt the pressure for things to go well, and blamed yourself if things didn't go as expected even if you are not really to blame?

Q. Do I feel responsible for other people's enjoyment of things?	Yes ☐	No ☐
Q. Do I blame myself when things go wrong?	Yes ☐	No ☐

Q. Have you noticed any of these examples of bearing all responsibility in the last week?

I must make sure that he/she has a good time.	Yes ☐	No ☐
It's my fault it went wrong.	Yes ☐	No ☐

Q. Have you noticed any other examples of bearing all responsibility?

✎ Write here the example(s) you noticed:

---

f) Making extreme statements and rules

Q. Do you make very strong statements or rules? Yes ☐ No ☐

Q. Do I make 'must', 'should' 'got to' or 'ought' statements to myself? Yes ☐ No ☐

Q. Do I use the words 'always', 'never' and 'typical' a lot? Yes ☐ No ☐

Q. Have you made any extreme comments or set yourself an impossible goal in the last week such as:

I'll never get better	Yes ☐	No ☐
I won't enjoy it so what's the point	Yes ☐	No ☐
Nothing will make any difference	Yes ☐	No ☐
It will be awful	Yes ☐	No ☐
I must get it completely perfect	Yes ☐	No ☐

Sometimes, this way of thinking is described as **black or white** or **all or nothing** thinking. This can worsen how you feel and unhelpfully alter what you do.

Q. Have you noticed any other example(s) of making extreme statements and rules?

✎ Write here the example(s) you noticed:

All of these types of thinking are examples of **extreme thinking**. Extreme thinking can have an **unhelpful** impact on how you feel and what you do.

Q. What is the impact of my altered thinking?

Extreme thoughts are unhelpful because of the impact on you and others of believing them.

1   What you think can affect how you feel emotionally

Altered thinking with negative and extreme thoughts can make you feel worse. If you are always thinking that other people don't like you or think you're no good, or you believe the future is really bleak, you are likely to quickly become disheartened and depressed.

Negative thinking ⟶ Lowered mood

2   What you think can affect how you feel physically

Negative and extreme ways of thinking can have a physical impact on you by making you feel physically unwell. Mental depression can cause physical feelings of low energy, sickness, or pain. Sometimes it can also cause a worsening of existing physical problems such as migraines.

Negative thinking ⟶ Altered physical symptoms

3   What you think can affect what you do

Negative thoughts may cause you to stop doing things that previously gave you a sense of pleasure or achievement, or to start doing things that actually worsen how you feel. For example, sometimes people experiencing depression may stop visiting friends and start drinking to try and block how they feel.

Negative thinking ⟶ Altered behaviour

Q. Overall, do the extreme and negative thoughts have an unhelpful effect on me?   Yes ☐   No ☐

Summary for Area 2

Having answered these questions:

Q. Overall, do I have problems in this area?   Yes ☐   No ☐

Area 3: Altered behaviour in depression

Learning from the past

What people think affects what they do. Think about how you have tried to deal with problems or feeling down in the past, to see if this can help you to identify effective ways of dealing with it now. This can help you to avoid repeating unhelpful ways of coping that haven't worked before.

Some changes of behaviour in depression can make matters worse, but others can help you feel better, for example working with a health care practitioner. There are two ways in which unhelpful behaviours may add to feelings of depression:

1 Stopping or reducing doing things which are fun or give a sense of achievement (e.g. meeting up with friends, doing hobbies and interests).

2 Starting to do activities, which quickly become unhelpful (e.g. beginning to drink to block how you feel, or choosing to isolate yourself).

To begin with, you will find out whether **reduced activity** is affecting your depression.

Altered behaviour 1: Reduced activity in depression

When you become depressed, it is normal to find it is difficult doing things. This is because of:

● low energy and tiredness ('*I'm too tired*').

● low mood and little sense of enjoyment or achievement when things are done.

● negative thinking and reduced enthusiasm to do things ('*I just can't be bothered*').

It can sometimes feel as though **everything is too much effort. A vicious circle of reduced activity** may result.

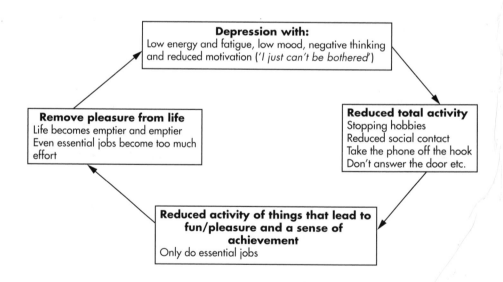

Figure 1.2 The vicious circle of reduced activity

A **vicious circle** occurs and this can keep the depression going. The good news is that once you have noticed if this is true for you, then you can begin to start working on regaining the pleasurable activities in a planned, step-by-step way. You will find out how to do this in a later workbook.

Now you can work out whether this problem is affecting you at the moment.

My reduced activity:

Please tick those areas you have noticed over the last week:

Stopping meeting friends	Yes ☐	No ☐
Reduced socialising/going out/joining in with others	Yes ☐	No ☐
Reduced hobbies/interests	Yes ☐	No ☐
Removal of pleasurable things from life	Yes ☐	No ☐
Life is becoming emptier	Yes ☐	No ☐

✎ Other (write in)

Altered behaviour 2: Unhelpful behaviour in depression

When somebody becomes depressed, it is normal for him or her to alter their behaviour to try and get better.

Helpful activities may include:

- talking to friends for support;
- reading or using self-help materials to find out more about the causes and treatment of depression;
- going to see their doctor or health care practitioner to discuss what treatments may be helpful for them;
- maintaining activities that give pleasure such as meeting friends etc.

Sometimes however, the person may try to block how they feel by using **unhelpful behaviours** such as:

- withdrawing into themselves and cutting themselves off from all their friends;

- using alcohol to block how they feel;

- neglecting themselves (e.g. by not eating as much);

- harming themselves as a way of blocking how you feel (e.g. self-cutting).

A vicious circle of unhelpful behaviours can result.

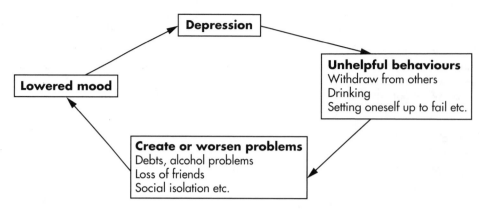

Figure 1.3. The vicious circle of unhelpful behaviour

My unhelpful behaviours

Please look at the following questions and **tick yes** if you have found yourself doing these things in the last week.

Q. Am I misusing alcohol to block how I feel?   Yes ☐   No ☐

Q. Am I misusing other substances such as illegal drugs?   Yes ☐   No ☐

Q. Am I becoming excessively clingy and dependent?   Yes ☐   No ☐

Q. Am I becoming very suspicious and demanding?   Yes ☐   No ☐

Q. Am I setting myself up to fail?   Yes ☐   No ☐

Q. Am I setting myself up to be let down or rejected?   Yes ☐   No ☐

Q. Am I trying to spend my way out of depression?   Yes ☐   No ☐

✎ Other (write in)

```



```

Q. Overall, does reduced activity have an unhelpful effect on me?   Yes ☐   No ☐

Summary for Area 3

Having answered these questions:

Q. Overall, do I have problems in this area?   Yes ☐   No ☐

Area 4: Altered physical feelings/symptoms in depression

In depression, a person may notice changes in their general well-being with:

- **Altered weight**

  Information: *Weight **loss** can occur as a result of reduced appetite. Sometimes weight **gain** can occur because of **comfort eating** and reduced activity since fewer calories are burned up. For some people, weight gain can cause them to feel even worse.*

- **Reduced energy**

  Information: *Low energy is a common problem and the person may feel tired all the time, and that they cannot do anything. As a result, in severe depression, things that previously would have seemed quite simple tasks such as getting dressed or washed or going out may become very difficult.*

Other common physical symptoms seen in depression are:

- **A reduced sex drive**

  Information: *Sex drive is often lost as part of the loss of pleasure and interest in things that is normal in depression. Often this is an area the person feels unwilling to talk about, but may lead to further upset if they are in a current relationship with a partner or spouse.*

- **Constipation**

  Information: *Constipation is common and is part of the physical slowing down of the body that occurs in depression. Eating lots of fruit and fibre, and drinking a reasonable amount of fluid can help this. Increases in activity levels such as by doing moderate exercise can also help overcome constipation. Sometimes, constipation is worsened by antidepressants. If you are unsure about this, please discuss it with your doctor.*

- **Symptoms of pain**

  Information: *If you already have problems such as arthritis or other physical problems, depression can often make it seem harder to cope. Pain can sometimes be an important symptom of depression. Depression may cause tension headaches, or contribute to chest or stomach pains such as those causing irritable bowel.*

- **Physical agitation**

  Information: *Depression can lead to a marked increase in symptoms of physical tension. This may mean that the person finds it difficult to sit still. They may become restless and feel forced to get up and walk around, being unable to settle.*

The following questions will help you to assess the impact of depression on your own body:

My physical symptoms of depression

Q. Which physical symptoms have you noticed over the last week?

Altered sleep symptoms:

- Wakening earlier than usual   Yes ☐   No ☐
- Difficulty getting off to sleep   Yes ☐   No ☐
- A disrupted sleep pattern   Yes ☐   No ☐

Altered appetite:

- An increased appetite   Yes ☐   No ☐
- A decreased appetite   Yes ☐   No ☐

Altered weight:

- Increased weight   Yes ☐   No ☐
- Decreased weight   Yes ☐   No ☐

Other symptoms:

- Reduced energy   Yes ☐   No ☐
- Reduced sex drive   Yes ☐   No ☐
- Constipation   Yes ☐   No ☐
- Symptoms of pain   Yes ☐   No ☐
- Physical agitation   Yes ☐   No ☐

✎ Other (write in):

Summary for Area 4

Having answered these questions:

Q. Overall, do I have problems in this area?   Yes ☐   No ☐

Area 5: Altered mood in depression

In depression, a person may notice changes in how they feel with:

Low mood

- **Information**: *Common terms that people use to describe low mood include depression, or feeling low/sad/blue/upset/down/miserable/fed up. Typically in severe depression the person feels **excessively** down and few if any things can pick them up from this feeling.*

Feeling worse (more depressed or lower in mood) first thing in the morning

- **Information**: *Mood that is worse in the morning and then improves as the day progresses can be a symptom of depression.*

A profound lack of enjoyment or pleasure in things

- **Information**: *Things that previously would have been fun or given a sense of pleasure now seem to lack any enjoyment. Sometimes the person may feel emotionless. In severe depression, almost nothing is enjoyed and it can seem that there are no emotions at all.*

Guilt

- **Information**: *In guilt, the person often feels terrible about letting themselves or others down. They feel bad because they believe they have failed against some legal or moral code or law.*

Worry, stress, tension or anxiety

- **Information**: *In worry, the person unhelpfully goes over things in their mind again and again. Doing this is not helpful because it doesn't help to solve the problems.*

Panic

- **Information:** *Sometimes levels of anxiety reach such a high level, that the person feels really panicky, very scared, even terrified, believing that something terrible is about to happen right now. It may lead to hasty measures such as stopping what they are doing and hurrying away. Such high levels of anxiety are **unpleasant but not dangerous**.*

Angry or irritable with yourself or with others

- **Information**: *Little things that normally wouldn't bother you seem to really irritate or upset you if you are feeling depressed. Anger tends to happen when you, or someone else, breaks a rule that you believe is important, or acts to threaten or frustrate you in some way.*

Ashamed or embarrassed at yourself or what you have done

- **Information**: *Feeling ashamed of yourself or your appearance can happen because you believe yourself to be inferior to others and fail to note your own achievements. You may feel embarrassed and think that others are judging you as having failed in some way.*

Suspicious and mistrusting of others

- **Information**: *When depression is present, sometimes this leads the person to doubt the motives of those around them, including close friends or relatives. At very high levels of depression, sometimes the person may lose all faith in others, and withdraw from possible important sources of support.*

KEY POINT

It is important to be very clear about the different emotional feelings you have. Try to notice changes in how you feel. These changes will often be linked with extreme thoughts, memories and ideas that are going through your mind at the time.

My altered emotional feelings

Which emotional changes have you noticed over the last week?

- Low or sad — Yes ☐ No ☐
- Feeling worse in the morning — Yes ☐ No ☐
- Reduced or no sense of pleasure in things — Yes ☐ No ☐
- Noticing no feelings at all — Yes ☐ No ☐
- Guilty — Yes ☐ No ☐
- Worried, stressed, tense or anxious — Yes ☐ No ☐
- Panicky — Yes ☐ No ☐
- Angry or irritable — Yes ☐ No ☐
- Ashamed — Yes ☐ No ☐
- Suspicious or mistrusting — Yes ☐ No ☐

Q. Overall, do I have any altered feelings? Yes ☐ No ☐

Emotions are an important and normal part of everyday life. Try not to be frightened by your feelings of depression. These emotions are a part of you and can help you to identify extreme and unhelpful thoughts that will be the targets for change. **Try to become aware of these thoughts and note them when you have a change in how you feel (your emotions).** Try to observe the thoughts as if you were a scientist trying to analyse the problem from a distance.

Summary for Area 5

Having answered these questions:

Q. Overall, do I have problems in this area? Yes ☐ No ☐

You have now finished your five areas assessment. Before you move on, please stop for a while and consider what you have learned. How does what you have read help you to make sense of your symptoms?

Q. How well does this assessment summarise how you feel?

Poorly ——————————————— Very well

0   10

A summary of how depression has affected you in the last week

The purpose of asking you to carry out the **five areas assessment** is not to demoralise you or to make you feel worse. Instead, by helping you consider how you are now, this can help you plan the areas you need to focus on to bring about change. The workbooks in the *Overcoming Depression* course can help you begin to tackle each of the five problem areas of depression.

Section 3   **The treatments of depression**

The main problem areas of depression are:

- current situations/events, relationship or practical problems;
- altered thinking;
- altered behaviour;
- altered physical symptoms;
- altered mood.

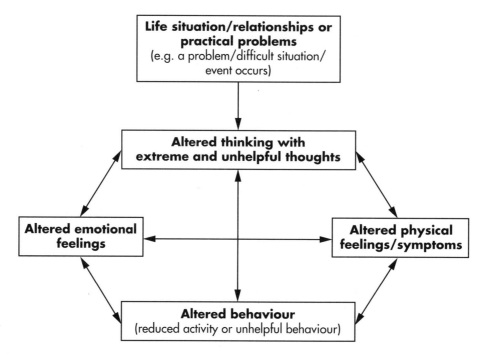

Figure 1.4 The five areas of depression

You have previously answered questions asking about each of these five areas. Go back and look at the symptoms you identified in each area to consider the impact of depression on you.

Links can occur between each of these areas. Because of this, aiming to **alter any** of these areas may help treat depression.

KEY POINT

By defining your problems, you have now identified **clear targets** to focus on. The key is to make sure that you do things **one step at a time**. A key to success is not to try to throw yourself into tackling everything at once. Slow steady steps are more likely to result in improvement than very enthusiastically starting and then running out of steam.

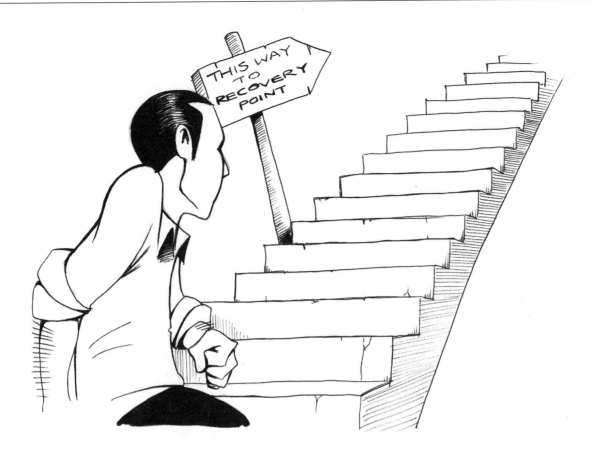

Choosing your targets for change

You may have tried all sorts of previous attempts to change, but unless you have a clear plan and stick to it, change will be very difficult. Planning and selecting which targets to try and change first is a crucial part of successfully moving forwards. By choosing which areas to focus on to start with, this also means that you are actively choosing at first **not** to focus on other areas.

Setting yourself **targets** will help you to focus on how to make the changes needed to get better. To do this you will need:

- **short-term** targets: thinking about changes you can make today, tomorrow and the next week;

- **medium-term** targets: changes to be put in place over the next few weeks;

- **long-term targets**: where you want to be in six months or a year.

The questions that you have answered in this workbook will have helped you to identify the main problem areas that you currently face. The *Overcoming Depression* course can help you to make changes in each of these areas.

The workbooks have been devised to be used either alone or as part of a complete course of ten workbooks. **Workbook 1** is designed to help you to identify your current problem areas. This will help identify which of the **workbooks 2–9** you need to read. Finally, you can summarise what you have learned and plan how to respond to any future feelings of depression by completing **workbook 10**. This will help you to reduce the chance that depression may affect you like this again.

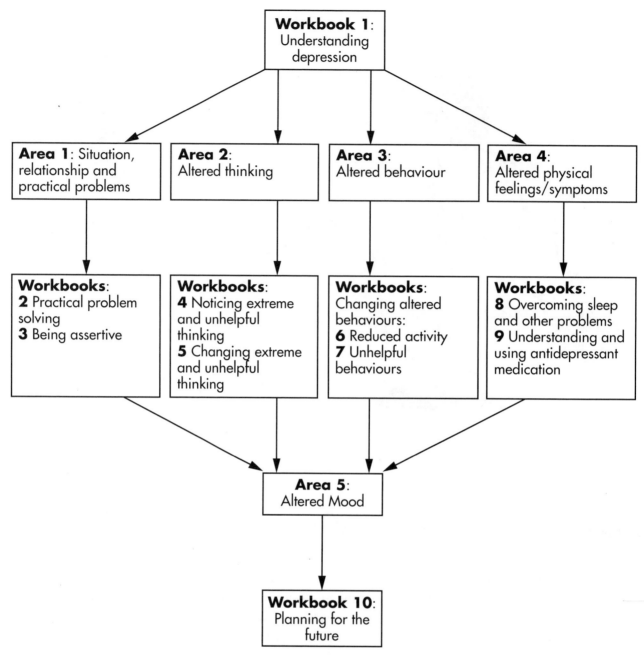

Figure 1.5 *Overcoming Depression*: course overview

The *Overcoming Depression* course

Workbook 1: *Understanding depression*

In this workbook you will learn about how depression alters your thinking and emotions, and leads to altered bodily symptoms and behaviour. This workbook will help you decide which of these areas you need to focus on changing and will help you decide which of the remaining workbooks you need to read. This is the workbook you are reading now.

Area 1: *Dealing with difficult situations, relationship and practical problems*

Workbook 2: *Practical problem solving*

In this workbook you will learn a step-by-step plan that you can use to deal with practical problems. It will provide you with the tools to tackle any practical problems that you face. This will help you to take more control of your life and the decisions that you make. By feeling more in control of your life, you will improve your confidence in yourself.

Workbook 3: *Being assertive*

Have you ever felt that no-one listens to you, and that other people seem to walk all over you, or have others commented that they feel that you always walk over them? You will find out about the difference between passive, aggressive and assertive behaviour and learn how to develop more balanced relationships with others where your opinion is listened to and respected, and you listen to and respect other people.

Area 2: *Changing extreme and unhelpful thinking*

Workbook 4: *Noticing extreme and unhelpful thinking*

What you think about yourself, others and the situations that occur around you, can alter how you feel and affect what you do. This workbook will help you to learn ways of identifying unhelpful or extreme ways of thinking. You will learn how to notice such thoughts and to understand the impact these have on how you feel and what you do.

Workbook 5: *Changing extreme and unhelpful thinking*

This workbook will teach you the important skill of how to challenge negative thinking. You will answer a series of questions that will help you change these thoughts. With practice this will help you begin to gain control of the extreme and negative thinking that is often a major problem in depression.

Area 3: *Changing altered behaviours*

Workbook 6: *Changing altered behaviours: reduced activity*

You will find out more about how altered behaviour keeps your depression going. You will learn ways of changing what you do in order to break the vicious circle of reduced activity.

Workbook 7: *Changing altered behaviours: unhelpful behaviours*

You will learn some effective ways of overcoming unhelpful behaviours such as drinking too much, reassurance-seeking and trying to spend your way out of depression.

Area 4: Physical symptoms and treatments in depression

Workbook 8: Overcoming sleep and other problems

Often when someone is depressed, they not only feel emotionally and mentally low, but they also notice a range of physical changes that are a normal part of depression. This workbook will help you find out about these common changes, and in particular will help you to deal with problems of poor sleep and low energy.

Workbook 9: Understanding and using antidepressant medication

When someone is depressed, sometimes their doctor suggests they take antidepressant medication. You will find out why doctors suggest this, and also learn about common fears and concerns that people have when first starting to take these tablets so that you can find out for yourself whether antidepressant medication may be helpful for you.

Area 5: Altered mood

The fifth and final area, low mood, will improve if you work at the other areas where you have problems (the altered thinking, behaviour, physical symptoms and the situations, relationships and practical problems that you face).

Once you feel better, the final workbook of the series can be read to help you to summarise what you have learned.

Workbook 10: Planning for the future

You will have learned new things about yourself and made changes in how you live your life. This final workbook will help you to identify what you have learned and help you plan for the future. You will be helped to devise your own personal plan to cope with future problems in your life so that you can face the future with confidence.

The work you do using the workbooks can supplement the help you receive from your doctor or other health care practitioners. Sometimes more specialist help is needed to help how you feel and your doctor may suggest that you see a trained specialist such as a psychologist, psychiatrist or a psychiatric nurse.

Use the following table to help you decide which workbooks are right for you to read. You may find it helpful to discuss this with your health care practitioner.

Workbook number	Plan to read	Tick when completed
Workbook 1: Understanding depression	✔	
Workbook 2: Practical problem solving		
Workbook 3: Being assertive		
Workbook 4: Noticing extreme and unhelpful thinking		
Workbook 5: Changing extreme and unhelpful thinking		
Workbook 6: Changing altered behaviours; reduced activity		
Workbook 7: Changing altered behaviours; unhelpful behaviours		
Workbook 8: Overcoming sleep and other problems		
Workbook 9: Understanding and using antidepressant medication		
Workbook 10: Planning for the future		

KEY POINT

In order to change, you will need to choose to try to **apply** what you will learn **throughout the week**, and not just when you read the workbook or see your health care practitioner. The workbooks will encourage you to do this by sometimes suggesting certain tasks for you to carry out in the days after reading each workbook.

These tasks will:

● help you to put into practice what you have learned in each workbook;

● gather information so that you can get the most out of the workbook.

Practice has shown that you are likely to make the most progress if you are able to put into practice what you have learned throughout the week.

Summary

The workbook has covered:
● how to use the workbook;
● symptoms in depression;
● the five areas of depression: the situations, relationship and practical problems faced by the person, and the altered thinking, emotional and physical feelings and behaviour that occur in depression;
● the impact of depression on you; helping you carry out your own **five areas assessment**;
● the treatments of depression; using your own five areas assessment to target areas for change;
● a description of the workbooks that make up the *Overcoming Depression* course so that you can choose which workbooks will be most helpful for you to use.

Preparing for the next workbooks

You have already begun to identify important changes in what you think and do. In order to build on what you have learned, it would be helpful if you could **gather some information** over the next week.

Please can you:

- Read through the current workbook again and think in detail about **how** depression is affecting your thinking, emotional and physical feelings, and behaviour and **what** you want to change.
- Choose **two episodes** over the next week when you feel more upset or depressed. Use the pages that follow this section **to record the impact on your thinking, mood, behaviour, and body.** Try to generate a summary of your own depression on each of the five areas of depression (life situation, relationships and practical problems, altered thinking, feelings, physical symptoms and behaviour). Look back to the '*Walking down the street*' example to help you try this task.
- When you have done this, choose your first area to begin working on and slowly read the workbook(s) in that area over a week or two. Put into practice what you have read, and then move on to other areas that you want to cover, making sure you allow yourself time to cover each area before moving on. Try to continue to put into practice what you have learned as you read further workbooks.

If you have difficulties with this workbook, don't worry. Just do what you can. If you have found any aspects of this workbook unhelpful, upsetting or confusing, please can you discuss this with your doctor or health care practitioner.

The five areas assessment of depression

Situation 1: A time when I am upset

1   Situation, relationship or practical problem

2   **My altered thinking**

3   **My altered feelings/emotions**

4   **My altered behaviour**

5   **My altered physical symptoms**

The five areas assessment of depression

Situation 2: A time when I am upset

1   Situation, relationship or practical problem

2   My altered thinking

3   My altered feelings/emotions

4   My altered behaviour

5   My altered physical symptoms

My notes

....

....

....

....

....

....

....

....

....

....

....

....

....

....

....

....

....

....

....

....

....

....

....

....

....

....

My notes

....

Workbook 2
Practical problem solving

Dr Chris Williams

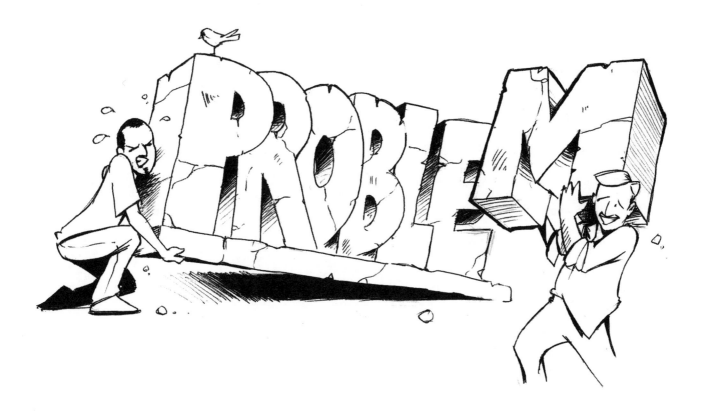

Overcoming Depression
A Five Areas Approach

Section 1   Introduction

In this workbook you will have a chance to find out about ways of tackling practical problems by learning about and practising a **practical problem solving approach.**

What are my practical problems?

First, think about the different situations, relationships and practical problems that you face:

Situation, relationship and practical problems

I have relationship difficulties (such as arguments) with:	Yes ☐	No ☐
✎ *(write in the person's name or initials)*		

```



```

I can't really talk to and receive support from my partner.	Yes ☐	No ☐
There is no one around who I can really talk to.	Yes ☐	No ☐
I feel stressed by the demands of looking after my children.	Yes ☐	No ☐
I have difficulties with money worries or debts.	Yes ☐	No ☐
I don't like where I live.	Yes ☐	No ☐
I am having problems with my neighbours.	Yes ☐	No ☐
I feel upset by my lack of a job.	Yes ☐	No ☐
I don't enjoy my job.	Yes ☐	No ☐
I have difficulties with colleagues at work.	Yes ☐	No ☐
✎ Other problems (**write in**)		

```



```

The key to the approach is *that it is not the events themselves that upset a person, but rather it is how they think about the events.* **However,** this does **not** mean that practical problems should be ignored. Instead the approach used in the *Overcoming Depression* course aims to help you to:
- Try to overcome practical problems using a problem solving approach.
- Try to alter any **unhelpful focus** on the problem (with negative and extreme thinking) by learning how to challenge extreme and unhelpful thinking. This is the focus of workbooks 4 and 5.

By approaching your practical problems one step at a time, it is possible to begin to tackle them. You can't deal with everything at once. In order to deal with them effectively, you need to prioritise and focus on changing just **one** area to begin with. This means that you must first try to put other problems to one side at the moment.

Think about and answer for yourself these questions:

Q. What might be the advantage of planning to change just one problem at first?

Write your answer here:

Q. What are the potential dangers of trying to change *everything* at once?

Write your answer here:

Section 2   Practical problem solving

The steps of problem solving include:
- approaching each problem separately in turn;
- defining the problem clearly;
- breaking down seemingly enormous and unmanageable problems into smaller parts that are then easier to solve;
- the need to approach the problem one step at a time.

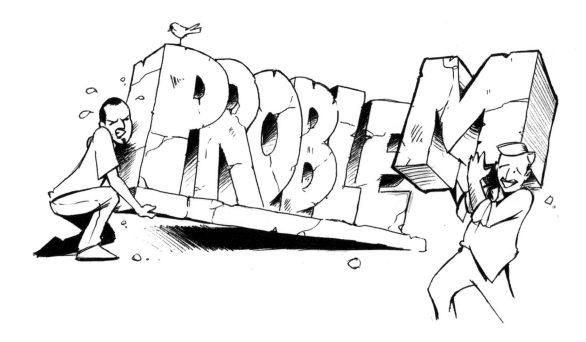

Problem solving is a logical process
By working through the seven steps outlined below you can learn an approach that enables you to solve your own problems.

Example
Paul is a 35 year old man who is currently feeling depressed. He has been off work and is now unable to pay his credit card bill this month because his income has reduced as a result of sick leave.

The seven steps to problem solving

Step 1: Identify and clearly define the problem as precisely as possible

> **Paul's problem:**
>
> *Not being able to pay my credit card bill this month.*
>
> Q. Is this a clear, focused problem?   Yes ✓   No ☐

Step 2: Brainstorm possible solutions

One problem that often faces people when they feel overwhelmed by practical problems is that they cannot see a way out. It can seem difficult to even start tackling the difficulty. One way around this is to try to step back from the problem and see if any other solutions are possible. This approach is called **brainstorming**.

- The more solutions that are generated, the more likely it is that a good one will emerge.
- Ridiculous ideas should be included as well even if you would never choose them in practice. This can help you adopt a **flexible** approach to the problem. What helpful ideas would others (e.g. family, friends) suggest?

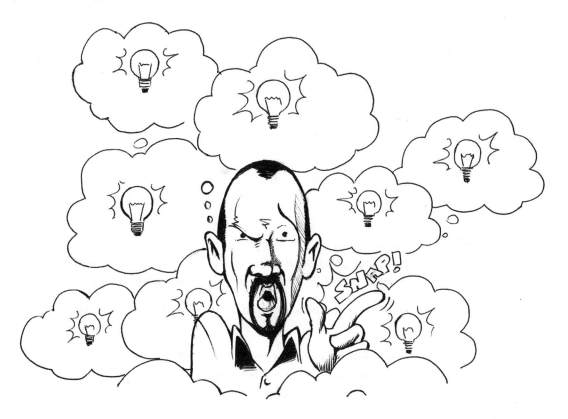

Paul's problem:

Possible options (including ridiculous ideas at first) are:

- *Ignore the problem completely - it may go away.*

- *Mug someone or rob a bank.*

- *Try to arrange a loan or overdraft from the bank and use this to pay off the bill.*

- *Pay off a very small part of the money (the minimum asked for).*

- *Switch my credit card payments to another credit card (one with a lower interest rate).*

- *Speak to a counsellor with skills in debt repayments.*

- *Speak to the credit card company to see if they will agree different re-payment terms.*

Step 3: Assess how effective and practical each potential solution is

Suggestion	Advantages	Disadvantages
Ignore the problem completely	*Easier in the short-term with no embarrassment.*	*The problems will worsen in the long-term. It will have to be tackled sometime.*
Mug someone or rob a bank	*It would get me some money.*	*It's unethical and wrong. I couldn't do it. I might be arrested. I couldn't harm someone else in this way. That's just ridiculous.*
Arrange a loan or overdraft with my bank	*It would allow me a better rate of interest than paying off the high rate on my credit card. I could also spread the payments over a longer time.*	*How would I do this? It would be scary seeing the bank manager. They may also say 'no'.*
Pay off the minimum payment possible	*Good short-term answer. It would prevent me defaulting the payments.*	*The debt wouldn't get any smaller, and the interest rates will make it larger and larger. I'll never be able to pay it off.*
Switch to a cheaper credit card	*This would be a lot cheaper. There are lots of good deals around with cheaper introductory rates.*	*I would need to look at the small print of the different agreements and complete all the paperwork.*
Speak to a debt counsellor	*I hear they can be very good.*	*I'd feel embarrassed talking to them. How do you contact them?*
Inform the credit card company and ask if they will agree different repayment terms	*It would provide the company with clear information. It's in their best interests for me to keep up the payments. They may be flexible and allow a repayment break at lower interest.*	*It seems quite scary to do this.*

Step 4: Choose one of the solutions

> This solution should be an option that fulfils the following two criteria:
>
> **a)** Is it helpful?   Yes ✓   No ☐
>
> **b)** Is it achievable   Yes ✓   No ☐

> **Paul's choice:**
>
> Paul decides on balance to arrange a bank loan or overdraft. This seems a reasonable solution. Other suggestions might also have worked, but this suggestion fulfils the two criteria above.

Step 5: Plan the steps needed to carry it out

Paul's plan:

I could phone my bank. I have the phone number on my bank statement. I'm quite nervous so I'm going to plan out what I am going to say in advance. I will phone up and ask to arrange a time to come in. I will tell them I am having problems repaying my credit card because I am off work sick. I will ask if I can come in to see someone in the afternoon because I feel better then. I think it's best if I also phone them in the afternoon. I'm more likely to get straight through to them then, and also I generally feel more confident after lunch.

Next, Paul needs to apply the *questions for effective change* to his plan to check how practical and achievable it is.

The *questions for effective change*

Is the planned solution one that: **Paul's plan:**

1   Will be **useful** for understanding or changing how I am?   Yes ✓   No ☐

2   Is a **specific task** so that I will know when I have done it?   Yes ✓   No ☐

3   Is **realistic**: is it practical and achievable?   Yes ✓   No ☐

4   Makes clear **what** I am going to do and **when** I am going to do it? Yes ✓   No ☐

5   Is an activity that won't be easily blocked or prevented by practical problems? Yes ✓   No ☐

Step 6: Do it!

Paul's plan

Paul phones up and arranges an appointment. When he goes to the bank, he feels quite scared. He predicts that the manager will humiliate him and turn his request down and that everyone will know what has happened.

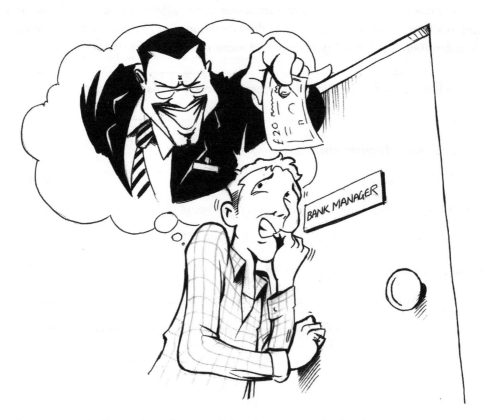

Paul decides to try to challenge these fears and decides to go to the bank anyway.

When he arrives at the bank, Paul is surprised to be met by a friendly bank assistant not the manager. She says that she is his personal account manager. She offers him a cup of tea, and they talk in a separate office so that their discussion is confidential. She tells him that this is a common problem. Because he has banked with them for several years and has a good banking record, she says there will be no problems in offering him a loan at a preferential rate. Paul agrees, and is happy with how things went. His fears were not correct. He was offered a loan. This is at a rate that he can afford.

Step 7: Review the outcome

Checklist:		
		Paul's review:
Q. Was the selected solution successful?	Yes ✓	No ☐
Q. Did it help pay off the credit card debt (the target problem)?	Yes ✓	No ☐
Q. Were there any disadvantages to using this approach?	Yes ☐	No ✓

Paul's review:

In this case, Paul's plan went smoothly. Even if there were any problems, he could have learned from them and used them to improve his next attempt to solve the problem.

The example used shows how the technique might be applied to this situation. However, it also works for **any** day-to-day difficulties. You now have the option of practising this approach:

Section 3 Putting what you have learned into practice

Think about how you can begin to tackle the problems you face in your own life.

Planning to overcome my practical problem

Step 1: Identify and clearly define the problem as precisely as possible

My problem: (please write in)

✎

> _(blank box)_

Q. Is this a clear, focused problem?   Yes ☐   No ☐

If no, re-write it so that it is clear and focused.

✎

> _(blank box)_

Step 2: Brainstorm possible solutions

- The more solutions that are generated, the more likely a good one will emerge.

- Ridiculous ideas should be included as well even if you would never choose them in practice. This can help you adopt a flexible approach to the problem. What helpful ideas would others (e.g. family, friends) suggest?

Brainstorming my problem:

Possible options (including ridiculous ideas at first) are:

✎

> _(blank box)_

Step 3: Assess how effective and practical each potential solution is

Suggestion	Advantages	Disadvantages

Try to create **as many** ideas as you can. If this proves difficult, try to think of some bizarre ideas first to help get the ideas flowing.

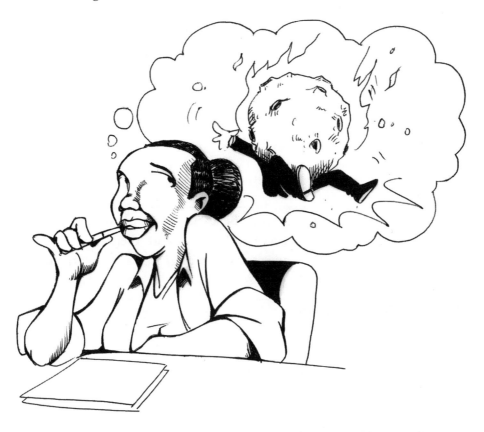

Try to **think broadly**. What helpful advice would a close friend or relative tell you? How could you look at the solutions facing you differently? Try to be creative in your answers. If you feel stuck, sometimes doing this task with someone you trust can be helpful.

Step 4: Choose one of the solutions

This solution should be an option that fulfils the following two criteria:

a) Is it helpful?   Yes ☐   No ☐

b) Is it achievable?   Yes ☐   No ☐

My choice:

✎

[ ]

Step 5: Plan the steps needed to carry it out

Write down the practical steps needed to carry out your plan. Try to be very specific in your plan so that you know what you are going to do, and when you are going to do it.

My plan:

✎

[ ]

This is **the key part** of the problem solving process. Be as precise as possible in your plan. Try to predict possible problems and work out how to avoid or deal with them.

Next, apply the *questions for effective change* to your plan to check how practical and achievable it is.

The questions for effective change

Is my planned task one that:

Q. will be useful for understanding or changing how I am?   Yes ☐   No ☐

Q. is a specific task so that I will know when I have done it?   Yes ☐   No ☐

Q. is realistic: is it practical and achievable?   Yes ☐   No ☐

Q. makes clear what I am going to do and when I am going to do it?   Yes ☐   No ☐

Q. is an activity that won't be easily blocked or prevented by practical problems? Yes ☐   No ☐

Step 6: Do it

What happened?

✎

Step 7: Review the outcome

Checklist

Q. Was the selected solution successful?   Yes ☐   No ☐

Q. Did it help deal with the target problem?   Yes ☐   No ☐

Q. Were there any disadvantages to using this approach?   Yes ☐   No ☐

Q. What have I learned from doing this?

Task

Write down any helpful lessons or information you have learned from what happened. If things didn't go quite as you hoped, try to learn from this. How could you make things different during your next attempt to tackle the problem?

My review:

✎

Conclusion

Problem solving is a technique that needs to be practised and you will improve your skills in this approach by using it. Try to learn from any mistakes and keep practising so that using this approach becomes second nature whenever you face a problem.

Putting what you have learned into practice

- Choose one or two problems only and start the seven step problem solving approach during the next 2 or 3 weeks.
- After a week of trying this, **then** read the final part of the workbook.

Section 4   **Review of your problem solving plan**

2.14

Q. Were you able to carry out your plan?   Yes ☐   No ☐

If no: Move back to the heading Planning to overcome my practical problem (section 3, pp 2.10).

If yes:

Q. How helpful was what you did in solving your problem?

Very unhelpful _____ Very helpful

                          0   10

If you noticed that your plan *was* helpful

This shows that you have gained by choosing to plan how to overcome your problem. By using this practical problem solving approach successfully, you have learned something important – that it is possible to change problems by approaching them one step at a time. By making slow, sure steps you will be able to boost your confidence and increase your sense of having the ability to deal with the problems you face. Think about how you can apply what you have learned over the next weeks.

If you noticed that your plan was *not* very helpful

Choosing realistic targets for change is important. Were you too ambitious or unrealistic in choosing the target you did? Sometimes a problem solving approach may be blocked by something unexpected that happens. Perhaps something didn't happen as you planned, or someone reacted in an unexpected way? Try to learn from what happened. How could you change how you approach the problem and continue to apply the *questions for effective change* to help you create a realistic action plan?

Q. How easy was it for you to complete the actions needed as part of the plan?

Very difficult_____ Very easy

0   10

If it was fairly easy to carry out the plan

If you found it easy to plan out and put into practice your problem solving plan, well done. This shows that you effectively planned out what you wanted to do. The best way to make a plan go smoothly is to have predicted possible problems, and clearly planned out what you are going to do at every stage.

If it was quite hard for you to do the task

When a person finds that their problem solving plan hasn't gone as smoothly as they would wish, it is often because they have:

- chosen a solution that is not very realistic or achievable (this is covered in steps 3 and 4 of the problem solving process).

- not planned out in enough detail every step they need to do in solving the problem (this is step 5 of the problem solving process).

Problem solving is a technique that needs to be practised and you will improve your skills in this approach by using it.

Workbook summary

In this workbook you have:

- Found out about ways of tackling practical problems by learning about and practising a **practical problem solving** approach.

Putting what you have learned into practice

Please can you continue to put into practice what you have learned over the next few weeks. Do not try to solve every problem all at once, but plan out what to do at a pace that is right for you. Discuss this with your health care practitioner if you are stuck or unsure what to do.

My notes

....

....

....

....

....

....

....

....

....

....

....

....

....

....

....

....

....

....

....

....

....

....

....

....

....

My notes

....

Workbook 3
Being assertive

Dr Chris Williams

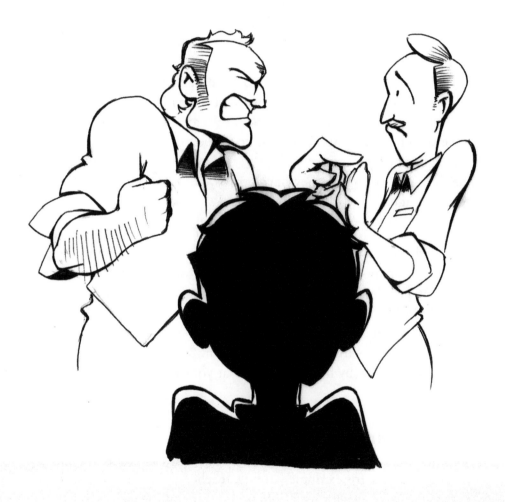

Overcoming Depression
A Five Areas Approach

Section *1*   **Introduction**

In this workbook you will:

- find out about the difference between passive, aggressive and assertive behaviour;
- learn about the rules of assertion and how you can put them into practice;
- practise assertive techniques in your own life.

What is assertiveness?

Assertiveness is being able to stand up for yourself, making sure your opinions and feelings are considered and not letting other people always get their way. It is **not** the same as aggressiveness. You can be assertive without being forceful or rude. Instead, it is stating clearly what you expect and insisting that your rights are considered.

Assertion is a skill that can be learnt. It is a way of communicating and behaving with others that helps the person to become more confident and aware of themselves.

At some time in each of our lives, however confident we are, we will find it difficult to deal with certain situations we encounter. Examples of these could be:

- dealing with unhelpful shop assistants;
- asking someone to return something they have borrowed;
- reacting to angry colleagues at work;
- communicating our feelings to our spouse, partner, family or friends.

Often in life we deal with these situations by losing our temper, by saying nothing or by giving in. This may leave us feeling unhappy, angry, out of control and still may not actually solve the problem. This tendency that many people have to react in either an unassertive or an aggressive way may become even more of a problem if they become depressed. The loss of confidence and self-worth that is common in depression may make the person more likely to **give in** to everyone around them, or in contrast become **very irritable** towards those around them. Both responses are unhelpful because they are likely to worsen how you feel (by being frustrated at yourself and others), and add to your problems.

Where does assertiveness come from?

As we grow up we learn to adapt our behaviour as a result of the things that happen to us. We model ourselves upon those around us, for example parents, teachers and our friends, and other influences such as television and magazines. If during this time our self-confidence is eroded, for example through being bullied or ridiculed at school or criticised within the family, then in our adult lives we may be more likely to react passively or aggressively in similar situations.

Although a person may have learned to react passively or aggressively in life, they can change and learn to become more assertive. You will now look at the effects of acting in an *aggressive* or a *passive* way, and then contrast this with the impact of *assertion*.

Elements of passive behaviour

Passive behaviour is **not** expressing your *feelings, needs, rights* and *opinions*. Instead there is an over-consideration for others' feelings, needs, rights and opinions.

Feelings   Bottling up your own feelings or expressing them in indirect or unhelpful ways.

Needs   Regarding the other person's needs as **more important** than your own. Giving in to them all the time.

Rights   The other person has rights but you do not allow yourself the same privilege.

Opinions   You see yourself as having little or nothing to contribute and the other person as always right. You may be frightened to say what you think in case your beliefs are ridiculed.

The aim of passive behaviour is to **avoid conflict** at all times and to **please others**.

Effects of passive behaviour

On you: short-term:

- reduction of anxiety;
- avoidance of guilt;
- martyrdom.

On you: long-term:

- continuing loss of self-esteem;
- increased internal tensions leading to stress, anger and worsened depression.

There are immediate positive effects of being passive but the longer lasting effects may be detrimental to your own health and cause others to become increasingly irritated by you and to develop a lack of respect for you.

Elements of aggressive behaviour

Aggression is the opposite of assertion. Aggression is expressing your own feelings, needs, rights and opinions with **no respect** for other people's feelings, needs, rights and opinions.

Feelings   Expressing your feelings in a demanding, angry and inappropriate way.

Needs   Your own needs are seen as being more important than others and theirs are ignored or dismissed.

Rights   Standing up for your own rights, but doing so in such a way that you violate the rights of other people.

Opinions   You see yourself as having something to contribute and see other people as having little or nothing to contribute.

The aim of aggression is to **win**, if necessary at the expense of others. Try to think of a time when someone else has been aggressive to you and ignored your opinions. How did it make you feel about them and yourself?

Effects of aggression

Aggression has both short-term and long-term consequences.

Short-term:

- release of tension;
- the person feels more powerful.

Long-term:

- feelings of guilt and shame;
- place responsibility for anger onto others;
- decreasing self-confidence and self-esteem;
- resentment in those around the aggressive person.

Although the short-term effects may be rewarding, the longer lasting effects of using aggression may be less beneficial and cause problems for the person and others.

Elements of assertive behaviour

In contrast to aggression and passivity, assertion is expressing your **own** feelings, needs, rights and opinions while maintaining respect for **other people's** feelings, needs, rights and opinions.

Feelings   When you are being assertive, you are able to express your feelings in a direct, honest and appropriate way.

Needs   You have needs that have to be met otherwise you feel undervalued, rejected, angry or sad.

Rights   You have basic human rights and it is possible to stand up for your own rights in such a way that you do not violate another person's rights.

Opinions   You have something to contribute irrespective of other people's views.

Assertion is not about winning, but it is concerned with being able to walk away feeling that you put across what you wanted to say. Try to think about a time when someone else has been assertive with you and respected your opinion. How did you feel about them and yourself?

About me – I felt: (write here):

About them – I felt: (write here):

The benefits of assertion

Assertiveness is an **attitude** towards yourself and others that is helpful and honest. In assertiveness you ask for what you want:
- directly and openly;
- appropriately, respecting your own opinions and rights and expecting others to do the same;
- confidently without undue anxiety.

You do not:
- violate people's rights;
- expect other people to magically know what you want;
- freeze with anxiety and avoid difficult issues.

The result is improved self-confidence in you and mutual respect from others.

The rules of assertion

All people have basic human rights that give us dignity as individuals. By not allowing your rights to be violated you are not being selfish but are maintaining your self-respect. As well as being aware of your own rights, if you respect other people's rights you have the foundation for assertive communication.

The rules of assertion

I have the right to:

1 **respect myself** – who I am and what I do.

2 **recognise my own needs as an individual** – that is separate from what is expected of me in particular roles, such as *'wife'*, *'husband'*, *'partner'*, *'son'*, *'daughter'*.

3 **make clear 'I' statements** about how I feel and what I think; for example, *'I feel very uncomfortable with your decision'*.

4 **allow myself to make mistakes**, recognising that it is normal to make mistakes.

5 **change my mind**, if I choose.

6 **ask for 'thinking it over time'**; for example, when people ask you to do something, you have the right to say *'I would like to think it over and I will let you know my decision by the end of the week'*.

7 **allow myself to enjoy my successes**, that is by being pleased with what I have done and sharing it with others.

8 **ask for what I want**, rather than hoping someone will notice what I want.

9 **recognise that I am not responsible for the behaviour of other adults.**

10 **respect other people** and their right to be assertive and expect the same in return.

Currently, how much do you believe each of these rules, and put them into practice?

The rules of assertion

I have the right to:	Do I believe this rule is true?		Have I applied this in the last week?	
1 Respect myself	Yes ☐	No ☐	Yes ☐	No ☐
2 Recognise **my own needs** as an individual independent of others	Yes ☐	No ☐	Yes ☐	No ☐
3 Make clear 'I' statements about how I feel and what I think; for example, *'I feel very uncomfortable with your decision'*	Yes ☐	No ☐	Yes ☐	No ☐
4 Allow myself to make mistakes	Yes ☐	No ☐	Yes ☐	No ☐
5 Change my mind	Yes ☐	No ☐	Yes ☐	No ☐
6 Ask for *'thinking it over time'*	Yes ☐	No ☐	Yes ☐	No ☐
7 Allow myself to enjoy my successes	Yes ☐	No ☐	Yes ☐	No ☐
8 Ask for what I want, rather than hoping someone will notice what I want	Yes ☐	No ☐	Yes ☐	No ☐
9 Recognise that I am not responsible for the behaviour of other adults	Yes ☐	No ☐	Yes ☐	No ☐
10 Respect other people and their right to be assertive and expect the same in return	Yes ☐	No ☐	Yes ☐	No ☐

It is possible to practise putting these rights into practice by using a number of assertiveness techniques.

'Broken record'

This is a useful technique and can work in virtually any situation. You rehearse what it is you want to say by **repeating over and over again** what it is you want or need. During the conversation, keep returning to your prepared lines, stating clearly and precisely exactly what it is you need or want. Do not be put off by clever arguments or by what the other person says. Once you have prepared the lines you want to say, you can relax. **There is nothing that can defeat this tactic**.

Example

Anne: *'Can I borrow £10 from you?'*

Paul: *'I cannot lend you any money. I've run out.'*

Anne: *'I'll pay you back as soon as I can. I need it desperately. You are my friend aren't you?'*

Paul: *'I cannot lend you any money.'*

Anne: *'I would do the same for you. You won't miss £10.'*

Paul: *'I am your friend but I cannot lend you any money. I'm afraid I've run out.'*

Remember:

● Work out beforehand what you want to say.

● Repeat your reply over and over again and stick to what you have decided.

This approach is particularly useful in:

● situations where your rights are being ignored;

● coping with clever, articulate people;

● situations where you may lose your self-confidence if you give in.

Saying 'no'

Many people find that saying 'no' seems to be one of the hardest words to say. We can sometimes be drawn into situations that we don't want to be in because we avoid saying this one simple word. The images we associate with saying 'no' may prevent us from using the word when we need it. We may be scared of being seen as mean and selfish, and of being rejected by others. Saying 'no' can be both important and helpful.

Q. Do I have problems saying 'no'?   Yes ☐   No ☐

If yes: try to practise saying 'no' by using the following principles:
● Be straightforward and honest but not rude so that you can make your point effectively.
● Tell the person if you are finding it difficult.
● Don't apologise and give elaborate reasons for saying 'no'. It is your right to say 'no' if you don't want to do things.
● Remember that it is better in the long run to be truthful than breed resentment and bitterness within yourself.

It may be that you have fears of how others may see or react to you if you do say 'no'. If these fears are not helpful or true, use the techniques that you have learned to challenge them. Remember, you cannot be responsible for the reactions of other adults, but you can be responsible for your own actions.

Scripting

Scripting involves planning out in advance in your mind or on paper exactly what you want to say in a structured way. This is a four-stage approach that covers:

- The **event**: the situation, relationship or practical problem that is important to you.

- Your **feelings**: how you feel about a situation or problem.

- Your **needs**: what you want to happen to make things different.

- The **consequences**: how making these positive changes will improve the situation for you and/or for others.

- **Event**: Say what it is you are talking about. Let the other person know precisely what situation you are referring to.

- **Feelings**: Express how the event mentioned affects your own feelings. Opinions can be argued with, **feelings cannot**. Expressing your feelings clearly can prevent a lot of confusion.

- **Needs**: People aren't mind readers. You need to tell them what you need. Otherwise people cannot fulfil your needs and this can lead to resentment and misunderstanding.

- **Consequences**: Tell the person that if they fulfil your needs, there will be a positive consequence for both of you. Be specific about the consequences.

A good way to begin to practise scripting is to **write down** what you want to say before you go into a situation. The 'event' and 'feelings' aspect of this can be used as a part of a broken record. Once you have engaged the person in discussion you can bring in the needs and consequences.

Example

Muriel: 'Hello, how are you?'

Joan: 'All right and you?'

Muriel: 'I saw Sandra yesterday. She said she was sorry to hear that I wasn't getting on with my neighbour. I told you about that in confidence. I didn't expect you to go round telling others.' **[Event]**

Joan: 'I thought Sandra was a good friend of yours. I didn't think you would mind. She asked how you were and said you seemed troubled. It seemed natural to tell her – why?'

Muriel: 'Sandra's okay but she has a tendency to discuss other people's problems with everyone she meets. I feel angry and upset that you have discussed this with her and let down by you as a friend.' **[Feeling]**

Joan: 'I didn't realise. I'm sorry.'

Muriel: 'I value our friendship and the fact that usually I can talk to you about things without you telling everyone else about it.'

Joan: 'Yes, I feel the same. I don't know what made me say anything to Sandra. She seemed genuinely concerned.'

Muriel: 'I'd like us to remain friends and to be able to share problems but I need to feel I can trust you.' **[Need]**

Joan: 'I won't make this mistake again. Let's not spoil our friendship over this.'

Muriel: 'We can stay friends but I would appreciate it if you didn't discuss my problems with others. Then we can both benefit from a friendship where we know a confidence will not be betrayed.' **[Consequence]**

Putting what you have learned into practice

Think about how you can be more assertive in your own life. If you recognise that a lack of assertiveness is a problem for you, try to:

- use one of the two assertiveness techniques during the forthcoming week.
- remind yourself about and put into practice the **rules of assertion.** This page can be torn out or photocopied so that you can carry it around with you, or put it in a prominent place (e.g. by your television or on a door or mirror) to remind you of these rules.
- after a week of trying this, **then** read the final part of the workbook.

The rules of assertion

I have the right to:

1 **respect myself** – who I am and what I do.

2 **recognise my own needs as an individual** – that is separate from what is expected of me in particular roles, such as 'wife', 'husband', 'partner', 'daughter', 'son'.

3 **make clear 'I' statements** about how I feel and what I think; for example, 'I feel very uncomfortable with your decision'.

4 **allow myself to make mistakes**, recognising that it is normal and acceptable to make mistakes.

5 **change my mind**, if I choose.

6 **ask for 'thinking it over time'**; for example, when people ask you to do something, you have the right to say 'I would like to think it over and I will let you know my decision by the end of the week'.

7 **allow myself to enjoy my successes**, that is by being pleased with what I have done and sharing it with others.

8 **ask for what I want**, rather than hoping someone will notice what I want.

9 **recognise that I am not responsible for the behaviour of other adults.**

10 **respect other people** and their right to be assertive and expect the same in return.

Section 2   **Review of your attempts to be assertive**

In the first part of the workbook, you learned that assertiveness is being able to stand up for yourself by making sure your opinions and feelings are considered. It is very different from being aggressive.

Elements of assertive behaviour

In contrast to aggression and passivity, assertion is expressing your **own** feelings, needs, rights and opinions with respect for **other people's** feelings, needs, rights and opinions.

Feelings   When you are being assertive, you are able to express your feelings in a direct, honest and appropriate way.

Needs   You have needs that have to be met.

Rights   You have basic human rights and it is possible to stand up for your own rights in such a way that you do not violate another person's rights.

Opinions   You have something to contribute irrespective of other people's views.

Assertion is not about winning, but it is concerned with being able to walk away feeling that you put across what you wanted to say.

Q. Were you able to act in an assertive way at some stage in the last week?

                                                        Yes ☐   No ☐

If yes: **were you able to respond**:

Q. Directly and openly?   Yes ☐   No ☐

Q. Appropriately?   Yes ☐   No ☐

Q. Respecting your own opinions and rights and expecting others to do the same?   Yes ☐   No ☐

Q. Overall, was the result improved self-confidence in you?   Yes ☐   No ☐

Review of the rules of assertion

The following table contains the *rules of assertion*. Look through them and then **please tick** those rules that you have, or could have, put into practice over the last week.

The rules of assertion

I have the right to:	Have I applied this in the last week?		*Could* I have applied this in the last week?	
1 Respect myself	Yes ☐	No ☐	Yes ☐	No ☐
2 Recognise my own needs as an individual independent of others	Yes ☐	No ☐	Yes ☐	No ☐
3 Make clear 'I' statements about how I feel and what I think. For example, '*I feel very uncomfortable with your decision*'	Yes ☐	No ☐	Yes ☐	No ☐
4 Allow myself to make mistakes	Yes ☐	No ☐	Yes ☐	No ☐
5 Change my mind	Yes ☐	No ☐	Yes ☐	No ☐
6 Ask for '*thinking it over time*'	Yes ☐	No ☐	Yes ☐	No ☐
7 Allow myself to enjoy my successes	Yes ☐	No ☐	Yes ☐	No ☐
8 Ask for what I want, rather than hoping someone will notice what I want	Yes ☐	No ☐	Yes ☐	No ☐
9 Recognise that I am not responsible for the behaviour of other adults	Yes ☐	No ☐	Yes ☐	No ☐
10 Respect other people and their right to be assertive and expect the same in return	Yes ☐	No ☐	Yes ☐	No ☐

If you could have been more assertive this week, but avoided putting the rules of assertion into practice, this shows that you need to continue to work on this area.

If you applied any of these rules of assertion in the last week, what was the impact on:

a) You?   Helpful ☐   Unhelpful ☐

b) Others?   Helpful ☐   Unhelpful ☐

Q. Did you fear that if you were assertive, it would go badly wrong?   Yes ☐   No ☐

If yes: Was this fear accurate and/or helpful?   Accurate ☐   Inaccurate ☐

     Helpful ☐   Unhelpful ☐

Often, one of the reasons why a person may avoid being assertive is that they **fear** what the consequences may be. They may mind-read that others will dislike them or reject them, or they may have catastrophic fears about the social consequences of assertion. As with most extreme fears, these fears are both untrue and inaccurate. One problem is that unless the person is able to identify and question their negative thoughts, they may **avoid** being assertive as a consequence. The very best way of challenging such thoughts is to **undermine** them by **choosing** to be assertive.

Summary

In this workbook you have:
- found out about the difference between passive, aggressive and assertive behaviour;
- learnt about the rules of assertion and how you can put them into practice;
- practised assertive techniques in your own life.

Putting into practice what you have learned

Re-read what you learned earlier in the workbook about the *broken record* and *scripting* approaches, and try to put them into practice during the next week. In particular, the scripting approach allows you to plan out how to be assertive in a particular situation and with a specific person. View this as a sort of action plan that can help you to both change how you are, and also learn something new about yourself and other people.

My notes

....

....

....

....

....

....

....

....

....

....

....

....

....

....

....

....

....

....

....

....

....

....

....

....

My notes

....

Workbook 4
Noticing extreme and unhelpful thinking

Dr Chris Williams

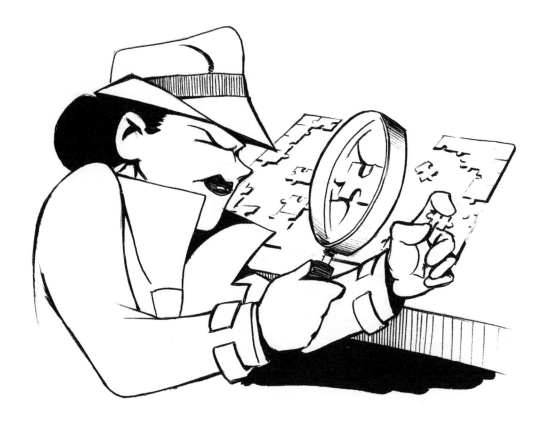

Overcoming Depression
A Five Areas Approach

Section *1* **Introduction**

This is the first of two workbooks that will help you find out about and begin to change unhelpfully altered thinking. In this workbook you will learn about:

● identifying unhelpful thinking;

● using a thought investigation worksheet to carry out an analysis of a time when your mood unhelpfully alters.

Revision

Unhelpful thinking styles

In order to be in a position to be able to challenge and change unhelpful and extreme thinking styles, it is important first of all to be aware of the common changes in thinking that can occur as part of depression. Depression can lead to one or more of the following unhelpful and extreme thinking styles:

Unhelpful thinking style	Typical negative thoughts	Tick if you have this thinking style
1 Bias against myself	I overlook my strengths I focus on my weaknesses I downplay my achievements I am my own worst critic	
2 Putting a negative slant on things (*negative mental filter*)	I see things through dark tinted glasses I tend to focus on the negative in situations	
3 Having a gloomy view of the future (make negative predictions/jump to the worst conclusion – *catastrophising*)	I make negative predictions about the future I predict that things will go wrong I predict that the very worst events will happen	
4 Negative view about how others see me (*mind-reading*)	I mind-read what others think of me I often think that others don't like me/think badly of me	
5 Bearing all responsibility	I take the blame if things go wrong I feel responsible for whether everyone else has a good time I take unfair responsibility for things that are not my fault	
6 Making extreme statements/rules	I use the words 'always', 'never' and 'typical' a lot to summarise things I make myself a lot of 'must', 'should' 'ought' or 'got to' rules	

All of these unhelpful thinking styles are examples of extreme thinking.

Why can extreme thinking be unhelpful?

In unhelpful thinking, thinking becomes biased and extreme and this has an impact on how you feel and on what you do. Typically, when these sorts of unhelpful thinking styles occur:

1 *Mood changes unhelpfully*: you may become depressed, upset, anxious, stressed or angry.
2 *Behaviour alters unhelpfully*: by either reducing what you do (reduced activity) or causing you to start unhelpful behaviours such as drinking too much to block how you feel. These changes lead to the *vicious circle of reduced activity* or the *vicious circle of unhelpful behaviours* referred to within the workbook *Understanding depression*.

The result is that these unhelpful thinking styles act to worsen how you feel and maintain your feelings of depression.

KEY POINT

The six unhelpful thinking styles are the main ways that thinking in depression can become extreme and unhelpful. Extreme thinking is unhelpful because it can worsen how you feel emotionally and also unhelpfully alter what you do. Thinking in extreme ways (sometimes called *black and white thinking*) means that you only look at part of the whole picture. Because of this, you will find out in the next workbook that extreme and unhelpful thinking is also often not true.

This workbook is designed to help you begin to practise ways of identifying extreme and unhelpful thinking. This is the key first step in beginning to change how you think so that you will be able to prepare for the next step of learning how to challenge these extreme thoughts. To do this, you will need to act like a thought detective by carrying out a **thought investigation** of the times when your mood alters unhelpfully.

Section 2 **Completing a thought investigation**

> **Hint**
>
> In order to identify extreme or negative thinking, try to watch for times when your mood suddenly changes (e.g. you feel sadder, or more anxious, upset or angry) then ask *'what went through my mind then'*?

The questions on the following pages will help you begin to work out how extreme thinking may affect how you feel and what you do. Try to **act like a detective** to piece together bit by bit the factors that led up to you feeling worse. An example of Muriel carrying out this process is provided later in the workbook.

Act like a detective

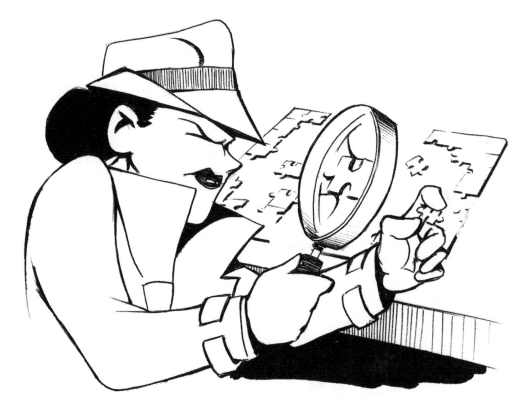

First, try to really **think yourself back into the situation** when your mood unhelpfully altered. Try to slow down how quickly you answer the questions on the next few pages so that you are as accurate as you can be in your thought investigation. Try to **stop, think and reflect** as you consider the five different areas that can be affected when mood alters.

The following questions will help you investigate for yourself the five areas that may be linked to unhelpfully altered mood by helping you to look in detail at:

1 the situation, relationship or practical problems that occurred, and to examine your:
2 altered thinking (such as extreme or unhelpful thinking styles);
3 altered feelings;
4 altered physical symptoms and also help you to consider any;
5 altered behaviour (such as reduced activity or starting to do unhelpful behaviours) that occurred.

Try to see how these different areas can link together to help you begin to understand how you feel during a time of altered mood.

Thought investigation. Events leading up to the mood change:

The situation, relationship or practical problem faced

4.5

---

a) The time:

Q. What time of day was it? It was . . . . o'clock.

---

b) The place:

Q. Where were you at the time? (Please tick)

I was:

- At home   Yes ☐   No ☐
- At work   Yes ☐   No ☐
- At the pub   Yes ☐   No ☐
- At a friend's house   Yes ☐   No ☐
- In a shop   Yes ☐   No ☐
- In town   Yes ☐   No ☐
- On a bus   Yes ☐   No ☐
- ✎ Other: I was . . .

---

c) The people. Who were you with?

You may have been alone, with only one or two people, or with many people.

Q. Were you alone?   Yes ☐   No ☐

If yes, skip to d. The events.

Q. Were you with a relative or relatives?   Yes ☐   No ☐

Q. Were you with a friend or friends?   Yes ☐   No ☐

Q. Were you with any other people?   Yes ☐   No ☐

✎ **If so, with whom?**

---

d) The current events/situation: What had upset you?

Think about the situation or events that led to your lowered mood. Had anything upsetting or stressful happened, for example an argument or an upsetting event?

I had been upset by:

- Something that was said   Yes ☐   No ☐
- How someone acted towards me   Yes ☐   No ☐
- Focusing on a practical problem I face   Yes ☐   No ☐
- A memory of something that had happened   Yes ☐   No ☐
- Worrying about the future   Yes ☐   No ☐
- Finally, had you had any alcohol to drink or used any drugs?   Yes ☐   No ☐
- ✎ Other events/situations

Altered emotional and physical feelings

a) Altered emotional feelings: consider how you felt emotionally at that time

When your mood altered, what emotional changes did you notice?

- I felt low and sad.   Yes ☐   No ☐
- I felt guilty and bad.   Yes ☐   No ☐
- I felt worried and stressed.   Yes ☐   No ☐
- I felt panicky.   Yes ☐   No ☐
- I felt angry or irritable about *myself*.   Yes ☐   No ☐
- I felt angry or irritable about *someone or something else*.   Yes ☐   No ☐
- I felt ashamed.   Yes ☐   No ☐
- I felt suspicious.   Yes ☐   No ☐
- I felt empty with no feelings at all.   Yes ☐   No ☐
- ✎ Other: I felt . . .

b) Altered physical feelings: what physical changes did you notice in your body?

When your mood altered, what physical changes did you notice?

- I felt that I had no energy/sapped of energy.   Yes ☐   No ☐

- I felt a feeling of pressure within me.   Yes ☐   No ☐

- I felt a feeling of heaviness inside.   Yes ☐   No ☐

- I felt tension in my arms or legs.   Yes ☐   No ☐

- I felt tension in my head or neck.   Yes ☐   No ☐

- I felt tension in my chest or stomach.   Yes ☐   No ☐

- I felt restless and wanted to move about.   Yes ☐   No ☐

- I felt slightly dizzy, spaced out or disconnected from things.   Yes ☐   No ☐

- I felt sick.   Yes ☐   No ☐

- I felt that I wasn't getting enough air into my lungs.   Yes ☐   No ☐

- I felt that my heart was speeded up.   Yes ☐   No ☐

✎ Other: I noticed . . .

Altered thinking: Identify and rate your belief in any thoughts that were present at the time

Think about what went through your mind at the time when your mood unhelpfully altered. Thoughts that are present when your mood alters are important because they are the thoughts that altered how you feel. They can be called *immediate thoughts*, because when they are present your mood *immediately* changed.

Q. What was going through your mind at that time?

At the moment your mood changed, what did you think about:

- Yourself?

- How others see you?

- What might happen in the future?

- Your own situation?

- Your own body, behaviour or performance?

- Were there any painful **memories** from the past?

- Did you notice any **images** or pictures in your mind? Images are an important type of thought and can have a powerful impact on how you feel.

To begin with, sometimes it can be difficult to notice these thoughts. With practice most people find that a number of negative or extreme thoughts are present at times when their mood unhelpfully alters.

✎ Write any immediate thoughts you noticed here:

Assessing my *belief* in the most powerful extreme and negative immediate thought

Choose the thought that seemed to have the greatest emotional impact on you

✎ Write it here:

Q. Overall, how much did you believe the most powerful thought at that time?

Make a cross on the line below to record how much you believed the thought.

Not at all believed _____ Completely believed

        0 per cent   50 per cent   100 per cent

Were any unhelpful thinking styles present when my mood unhelpfully altered?

Which of the unhelpful styles did you notice at that time? Read through the list and select those unhelpful thinking styles that were present.

Unhelpful thinking style	Typical negative thoughts	Tick here if you thought like this *at the time* your mood altered
Bias against myself	I overlook my strengths I focus on my weaknesses I downplay my achievements I am my own worst critic	
Putting a negative slant on things (*negative mental filter*)	I see things through dark tinted glasses I tend to focus on the negative in situations	
Having a gloomy view of the future (make negative predictions/Jump to the worst conclusion – *catastrophising*)	I make negative predictions about the future I predict that things will go wrong I predict that the very worst events will happen	
Negative view about how others see me (*mind-reading*)	I mind-read what others think of me I often think that others don't like me/think badly of me	
Bearing all responsibility	I take the blame if things go wrong I feel responsible for whether everyone else has a good time I take unfair responsibility for things that are not my fault	
Making extreme statements/rules	I use the words 'always', 'never' and 'typical' a lot to summarise things I make myself a lot of 'must', 'should' 'ought' or 'got to' rules	

The impact of the immediate thoughts on your behaviour

Consider the impact of any extreme thinking on your behaviour and how this affected you and others.

---

a) My reduced activity

When your mood altered, what changes occurred in what you said or did at the time?

Q. I reduced my activity levels when I felt like this. Yes ☐ No ☐

Q. I avoided doing a planned activity as a result. Yes ☐ No ☐

Q. I chose to avoid talking to or meeting anyone. Yes ☐ No ☐

Q. I decided not to go out. Yes ☐ No ☐

✎ Other: I . . .

---

b) My unhelpful behaviours

When your mood altered, did you do anything differently because of what happened?

Q. I became excessively clingy and dependent. Yes ☐ No ☐

Q. I became very suspicious and demanding. Yes ☐ No ☐

Q. I did something that set me up to fail. Yes ☐ No ☐

Q. I did something that set me up to be let down or rejected. Yes ☐ No ☐

Q. I had a drink to block how I felt. Yes ☐ No ☐

Q. I chose to misuse other tablets or used illegal drugs. Yes ☐ No ☐

Q. I did something to hurt myself such as cutting myself. Yes ☐ No ☐

✎ Other: . . .

Q. What was the impact of these unhelpful thinking styles on how I felt and what I did?

Extreme thoughts can unhelpfully change how you feel so that you feel more disheartened and depressed.

What you think can worsen how you feel emotionally

Extreme thinking ——————➤ Lowered mood

Q. What was the impact of the immediate thoughts on how you felt at the time your mood altered?

Helpful ☐   Unhelpful ☐

Extreme thoughts may also cause you to stop doing things that previously gave you a sense of pleasure or achievement, or to start doing things that actually worsen how you feel.

What you think can affect what you do

Extreme thinking ——————➤ reduced activity or unhelpful behaviours

Q. What was the impact of the immediate thoughts on what you did at the time your mood altered?

Helpful ☐   Unhelpful ☐

Overall, did extreme and negative thought(s) have an unhelpful effect on you?

Yes ☐   No ☐

If a thought shows one of the unhelpful thinking styles, and also has an unhelpful impact on you, then you have identified an example of an extreme and unhelpful thought. These are the sorts of thoughts that you will learn to challenge in workbook 5 (*Changing extreme and unhelpful thinking*).

Summary of my thought investigation of a time when my mood changed

Now that you have finished, re-read your answers in your thought investigation. As you do this, try to apply what you know about the *five areas assessment* model to see how each of these areas might have played a part in helping you understand how you feel.

The five areas assessment model

The five areas model shows that **what a person thinks** about a situation or problem may **affect how they feel** physically and emotionally, and also may lead them to alter **what they do** (altered behaviour).

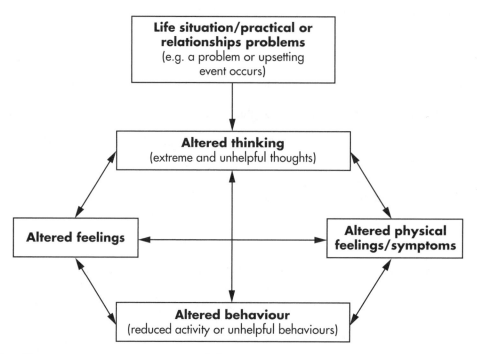

Figure 4.1 The five areas assessment model

At first, many people find it can be quite difficult to notice unhelpful thinking styles. Carrying out this sort of **thought investigation** can help you to begin to practise how to do this so that over time you find that this process becomes easier. The best way of becoming aware of your extreme and unhelpful thinking is to begin to try to notice times when your mood unhelpfully alters (e.g. at times when you feel upset), and then to ask '*What is going through my mind right now?*'

Practising thought investigation

A **thought investigation worksheet** has been produced to help you to practise this process of carrying out a thought investigation whenever your mood unhelpfully alters. The thought investigation worksheet on the next page shows a person called Muriel completing her own thought investigation using the worksheet. Muriel is a fifty-five year old woman who lives by herself. She is feeling depressed, and has reduced her activities at home and with other people, and asked her sister Mary not to visit her because she worries what she will think of her.

Example of Muriel completing her thought investigation worksheet: identifying extreme and unhelpful thinking

1 Situation/relationship or practical problem when your mood altered	2 Altered emotional and physical feelings	3 What immediate thoughts are present at the time?	4 What unhelpful thinking style(s) occur?	5 Impact of the immediate thought(s)
Think in detail: Where am I, what am I doing? Consider: ● **The time**: What time of day is it? ● **The place**: Where am I? ● **The people**: Who is present? Who am I with? ● **The events**: What has been said/What events happened?	Am I ● Low or sad? Guilty? ● Worried, tense, anxious or panicky? ● Angry or irritable? ● Ashamed or suspicious? **a)** State the feelings clearly. Try to be as precise as possible. If more than one feeling occurs, underline the most powerful feeling. **b)** How powerful is this feeling (0–100%)? **c)** Note down any strong physical sensations you notice.	What is going through my mind? How do I see: ● Myself/How others see me? ● The current events/situation. ● What might happen in the future? ● My own body, behaviour or performance? ● Any memories or images? **a)** State the thought(s) clearly. Try to be as precise as possible. If more than one thought occurs, underline the most powerful thought. **b)** Rate how strongly you believe the most powerful thought at the time (0–100%).	1 Bias against myself. 2 Putting a negative slant on things (negative mental filter). 3 Having a gloomy view of the future/jumping to the worst conclusion. 4 Negative view about how others see me (mind-reading). 5 Bearing all responsibility. 6 Making extreme statements/rules, e.g. using *must, should, ought, always,* and *never* statements. If any of the styles are present, you have identified an **extreme** thought.	**a) What did I do differently?** Consider any: ● Reduced activity. ● Unhelpful behaviours. **b)** What was the impact on: ● Myself? ● My view of others? ● How I felt? ● What I said? ● What I did? ● Overall, was the impact helpful or **unhelpful?** If there is an unhelpful impact, you have identified an **unhelpful** thought.
Situation: *10am at home. My sister Mary came by unexpectedly*	**a) My feelings:** *I felt low and sad. I felt ashamed.* **b) Powerfulness:** *0–100 % = 80 %* **c) Physical sensations:** *I blushed and felt hot*	**My immediate thought:** **a)** ✎ State the thought(s) clearly. *Oh no, I always look awful. She'll think I'm not coping.* If you have noticed more than one thought, **underline** the most powerful thought. **b)** ✎ Rate your belief in the most powerful thought at the time: 0% 100% ⊢———×———⊣	**Which thinking styles are present?** (please state numbers or types) ✎ No(s): *1, 3, 6*	**a) What did I do differently?** *I acted quite flustered* *I avoided eye contact.* *I made an excuse after ten minutes and told her I had to go to a doctor's appointment.* **b)** Overall, is it **helpful** or **unhelpful** for me to believe the thought? Helpful ☐ Unhelpful ✓

When you have read this, try to complete your own worksheet on several occasions each day for the next few days to practise this skill. You will find some blank practice worksheets at the back of this workbook. Please copy these out or photocopy them if you require further sheets.

Getting the most from the thought investigation worksheet

To get the most from the worksheet:

- Practise completing the worksheet whenever you notice your mood unhelpfully altering. With practice you will find it easier to identify your extreme thinking.

- Try to fill the worksheet in as soon as possible after you notice your mood change.

- If you cannot fill it in immediately, try to think yourself back into the situation so that you are as clear as possible in your answer.

KEY POINTS

- Noticing changes in your mood can be a helpful way of identifying extreme and unhelpful thinking.

- If a thought shows one or more of the unhelpful thinking styles, and has an unhelpful impact on how you feel or what you do, then you have identified an example of an extreme and an unhelpful thought. These are the sort of thoughts that are identified in **columns 4 and 5 of the thought investigation worksheet** and which will be the focus for change in the next workbook.

In the second workbook on this area, *Changing extreme and unhelpful thinking*, you will see that the worksheet has a second side that will help you to begin to challenge extreme and unhelpful thinking. For the time being, try to get used to using just the first side only as you practise carrying out a thought investigation. When you feel confident in doing this, you should move on to the next workbook, *Changing extreme and unhelpful thinking*.

Section 3 **Workbook summary**

In this workbook, you have learned about:

● identifying unhelpful thinking;

● using a thought investigation worksheet to carry out an analysis of a time when your mood unhelpfully alters.

Putting into practice what you have learned

You have already begun to identify important changes in what you think and do. You will build on this in workbook 5 *Changing extreme and unhelpful thinking*. In order to help prepare for this, it would be helpful if you could practise what you have learned over the next week. Please can you:

> ● Use the thought investigation worksheet to carry out a thought investigation on **four** occasions when your mood unhelpfully alters.
>
> ● **Stop and think** which unhelpful thinking style(s) you noticed during these times and **reflect** on the helpfulness and accuracy of the thoughts.
>
> ● Begin to ask yourself, *are the thoughts actually **true**?* How could I see things more helpfully and accurately – in a less extreme way?
>
> If you have difficulties with this, don't worry. Just do what you can and discuss any problems with your health care practitioner.

Practice 1 Thought investigation worksheet: identifying extreme and unhelpful thinking

1 Situation/relationship or practical problem when your mood altered.	2 Altered emotional and physical feelings	3 What immediate thoughts are present at the time?	4 What unhelpful thinking style(s) occur?	5 Impact of the immediate thought(s)
Think in detail: Where am I, what am I doing? Consider: ● **The time**: What time of day is it? ● **The place**: Where am I? ● **The people**: Who is present? Who am I with? ● **The events**: What has been said/What events happened?	Am I ● Low or sad? Guilty? ● Worried, tense, anxious or panicky? ● Angry or irritable? ● Ashamed or suspicious? **a)** State the feelings clearly. Try to be as precise as possible. If more than one feeling occurs, underline the most powerful feeling. **b)** How powerful is this feeling (0–100 per cent)? **c)** Note down any strong physical sensations you notice.	What is going through my mind? How do I see: ● Myself, How others see me? ● The current events/situation. ● What might happen in the future? ● My own body, behaviour or performance? ● Any memories or images? **a)** State the thought(s) clearly. Try to be as precise as possible. If more than one thought occurs, underline the most powerful thought. **b)** Rate how strongly you believe the most powerful thought at the time (0–100%).	1 Bias against myself. 2 Putting a negative slant on things (negative mental filter). 3 Having a gloomy view of the future/ jumping to the worst conclusion. 4 Negative view about how others see me (mind-reading). 5 Bearing all responsibility. 6 Making extreme statements/rules, e.g. using *must, should, ought, always,* and *never* statements. If any of the styles are present, you have identified an **extreme** thought.	**a)** What did I do differently? Consider any: ● Reduced activity. ● Unhelpful behaviours. **b)** What was the impact on: ● Myself? ● My view of others? ● How I felt? ● What I said? ● What I did? ● Overall, was the impact helpful or unhelpful? If there is an unhelpful impact, you have identified an **unhelpful** thought.
Situation:	**a) My feelings:** **b) Powerfulness:** 0–100% = **c) Physical sensations:**	**My immediate thought(s):** **a)** ✎ State the thought(s) clearly. If you have noticed more than one thought, **underline** the most powerful thought: **b)** ✎ Rate your belief in the most powerful thought at the time: 0% ⎯⎯⎯⎯⎯ 100%	**Which thinking styles are present?** (please state numbers or types) ✎ No(s):	**a)** What did I do differently? **b)** Overall, is it **helpful** or **unhelpful** for me to believe the thought? Helpful ☐ Unhelpful ☐

Practice 2 Thought investigation worksheet: identifying extreme and unhelpful thinking

1 Situation/relationship or practical problem when your mood altered.	2 Altered emotional and physical feelings	3 What immediate thoughts are present at the time?	4 What unhelpful thinking style(s) occur?	5 Impact of the immediate thought(s)
Think in detail: Where am I, what am I doing? Consider: ● **The time**: What time of day is it? ● **The place**: Where am I? ● **The people**: Who is present? Who am I with? ● **The events**: What has been said/What events happened?	**a) My feelings**: Am I ● Low or sad? Guilty? ● Worried, tense, anxious or panicky? ● Angry or irritable? ● Ashamed or suspicious? **a)** State the feelings clearly. Try to be as precise as possible. If more than one feeling occurs, <u>underline</u> the most powerful feeling. **b)** How powerful is this feeling (0–100%)? **c)** Note down any strong physical sensations you notice.	What is going through my mind? How do I see: ● Myself, How others see me? ● The current events/situation. ● What might happen in the future? ● My own body, behaviour or performance? ● Any memories or images? **a)** State the thought(s) clearly. Try to be as precise as possible. If more than one thought occurs, <u>underline</u> the most powerful thought. **b)** Rate how strongly you believe the most powerful thought at the time (0–100%).	1 Bias against myself. 2 Putting a negative slant on things (negative mental filter). 3 Having a gloomy view of the future/ jumping to the worst conclusion. 4 Negative view about how others see me (mind-reading). 5 Bearing all responsibility. 6 Making extreme statements/rules, e.g. using *must, should, ought, always, and never* statements. If any of the styles are present, you have identified an **extreme** thought.	**a)** What did I do differently? Consider any: ● Reduced activity. ● Unhelpful behaviours. **b)** What was the impact on: ● Myself? ● My view of others? ● How I felt? ● What I said? ● What I did? ● Overall, was the impact helpful or unhelpful? If there is an unhelpful impact, you have identified an **unhelpful** thought.
Situation:	**a) My feelings**: **b) Powerfulness**: 0–100% = **c) Physical sensations**:	**My immediate thought(s)**: **a)** ✎ State the thought(s) clearly. If you have noticed more than one thought, **underline** the most powerful thought. **b)** ✎ Rate your belief in the most powerful thought at the time: 0% 100%	**Which thinking styles are present?** (please state numbers or types) ✎ No(s):	**a)** What did I do differently? **b)** Overall, is it **helpful** or **unhelpful** for me to believe the thought? Helpful ☐ Unhelpful ☐

Practice 3 Thought investigation worksheet: identifying extreme and unhelpful thinking

1 Situation/relationship or practical problem when your mood altered.	2 Altered emotional and physical feelings	3 What immediate thoughts are present at the time?	4 What unhelpful thinking style(s) occur?	5 Impact of the immediate thought(s)
Think in detail: Where am I, what am I doing? Consider: ● **The time**: What time of day is it? ● **The place**: Where am I? ● **The people**: Who is present? Who am I with? ● **The events**: What has been said/What events happened?	**Am I** ● Low or sad? Guilty? ● Worried, tense, anxious or panicky? ● Angry or irritable? ● Ashamed or suspicious? **a)** State the feelings clearly. Try to be as precise as possible. If more than one feeling occurs, underline the most powerful feeling. **b)** How powerful is this feeling? (0–100%) **c)** Note down any strong physical sensations you notice.	What is going through my mind? How do I see: ● Myself, How others see me? ● The current events/situation. ● What might happen in the future? ● My own body, behaviour or performance? ● Any memories or images? **a)** State the thought(s) clearly. Try to be as precise as possible. If more than one thought occurs, underline the most powerful thought. **b)** Rate how strongly you believe the most powerful thought at the time (0–100%).	1 Bias against myself. 2 Putting a negative slant on things (negative mental filter). 3 Having a gloomy view of the future/ jumping to the worst conclusion. 4 Negative view about how others see me (mind-reading). 5 Bearing all responsibility. 6 Making extreme statements/rules, e.g. using *must, should, ought, always,* and *never* statements. If any of the styles are present, you have identified an **extreme** thought.	**a)** What did I do differently? Consider any: ● Reduced activity. ● Unhelpful behaviours. **b)** What was the impact on: ● Myself? ● My view of others? ● How I felt? ● What I said? ● What I did? ● Overall, was the impact helpful or unhelpful? If there is an unhelpful impact, you have identified an **unhelpful** thought.
Situation:	**a) My feelings:** **b) Powerfulness:** 0–100% = **c) Physical sensations:**	**My immediate thought(s):** **a)** ✎ State the thought(s) clearly. If you have noticed more than one thought, **underline** the most powerful thought. **b)** ✎ Rate your belief in the most powerful thought at the time: 0% 100%	**Which thinking styles are present?** (please state numbers or types) ✎ No(s):	**a)** What did I do differently? **b)** Overall, is it **helpful** or **unhelpful** for me to believe the thought? Helpful ☐ Unhelpful ☐

Practice 4 Thought investigation worksheet: identifying extreme and unhelpful thinking

1 Situation/relationship or practical problem when your mood altered.	2 Altered emotional and physical feelings	3 What immediate thoughts are present at the time?	4 What unhelpful thinking style(s) occur?	5 Impact of the immediate thought(s)
Think in detail: Where am I, what am I doing? Consider: • **The time**: What time of day is it? • **The place**: Where am I? • **The people**: Who is present? Who am I with? • **The events**: What has been said/What events happened?	Am I • Low or sad? Guilty? • Worried, tense, anxious or panicky? • Angry or irritable? • Ashamed or suspicious? **a)** State the feelings clearly. Try to be as precise as possible. If more than one feeling occurs, underline the most powerful feeling. **b)** How powerful is this feeling (0–100%)? **c)** Note down any strong physical sensations you notice.	What is going through my mind? How do I see: • Myself, How others see me? • The current events/situation. • What might happen in the future? • My own body, behaviour or performance? • Any memories or images? **a)** State the thought(s) clearly. Try to be as precise as possible. If more than one thought occurs, underline the most powerful thought. **b)** Rate how strongly you believe the most powerful thought at the time (0–100%).	1 Bias against myself. 2 Putting a negative slant on things (negative mental filter). 3 Having a gloomy view of the future/ jumping to the worst conclusion. 4 Negative view about how others see me (mind-reading). 5 Bearing all responsibility. 6 Making extreme statements/rules, e.g. using *must, should, ought, always,* and *never* statements. If any of the styles are present, you have identified an **extreme** thought.	**a)** What did I do differently? Consider any: • Reduced activity. • Unhelpful behaviours. **b)** What was the impact on: • Myself? • My view of others? • How I felt? • What I said? • What I did? • Overall, was the impact helpful or unhelpful? If there is an unhelpful impact, you have identified an **unhelpful** thought.
Situation:	**a) My feelings:** **b) Powerfulness:** 0–100% = **c) Physical sensations:**	**My immediate thought(s):** **a)** State the thought(s) clearly. If you have noticed more than one thought, **underline** the most powerful thought. **b)** Rate your belief in the most powerful thought at the time: 0%　　　　100%	**Which thinking styles are present?** (please state numbers or types) No(s):	**a)** What did I do differently? **b)** Overall, is it **helpful** or **unhelpful** for me to believe the thought? Helpful ☐ Unhelpful ☐

Thought investigation worksheet: identifying extreme and unhelpful thinking

1 Situation/relationship or practical problem when your mood altered.	2 Altered emotional and physical feelings	3 What immediate thoughts are present at the time?	4 What unhelpful thinking style(s) occur?	5 Impact of the immediate thought(s)
Think in detail: Where am I, what am I doing? Consider: ● **The time**: What time of day is it? ● **The place**: Where am I? ● **The people**: Who is present? Who am I with? ● **The events**: What has been said/What events happened?	Am I ● Low or sad? Guilty? ● Worried, tense, anxious or panicky? ● Angry or irritable? ● Ashamed or suspicious? **a)** State the feelings clearly. Try to be as precise as possible. If more than one feeling occurs, underline the most powerful feeling. **b)** How powerful is this feeling (0–100%)? **c)** Note down any strong physical sensations you notice.	What is going through my mind? How do I see: ● Myself, How others see me? ● The current events/situation. ● What might happen in the future? ● My own body, behaviour or performance? ● Any memories or images? **a)** State the thought(s) clearly. Try to be as precise as possible. If more than one thought occurs, underline the most powerful thought. **b)** Rate how strongly you believe the most powerful thought at the time (0–100%).	1 Bias against myself. 2 Putting a negative slant on things (negative mental filter). 3 Having a gloomy view of the future/ jumping to the worst conclusion. 4 Negative view about how others see me (mind-reading). 5 Bearing all responsibility. 6 Making extreme statements/rules, e.g. using *must, should, ought, always,* and *never* statements. If any of the styles are present, you have identified an **extreme** thought.	**a)** What did I do differently? Consider any: ● Reduced activity. ● Unhelpful behaviours. **b)** What was the impact on: ● Myself? ● My view of others? ● How I felt? ● What I said? ● What I did? ● Overall, was the impact helpful or unhelpful? If there is an unhelpful impact, you have identified an **unhelpful** thought.
Situation:	**a) My feelings:** **b) Powerfulness:** 0–100% = **c) Physical sensations:**	**My immediate thought(s):** **a)** ✐ State the thought(s) clearly. If you have noticed more than one thought, **underline** the most powerful thought. **b)** ✐ Rate your belief in the most powerful thought at the time: 0% 100%	**Which thinking styles are present?** (please state numbers or types) ✐ No(s):	**a)** What did I do differently? **b)** Overall, is it **helpful** or **unhelpful** for me to believe the thought? Helpful ☐ Unhelpful ☐

My notes

....

© 2001 Dr C. J. Williams and University of Leeds Innovations Ltd. (ULIS)   4.21

....

....

....

....

....

....

....

....

....

....

....

....

....

....

....

....

....

....

....

....

....

My notes

....

Workbook 5

Changing extreme
and unhelpful thinking

Dr Chris Williams

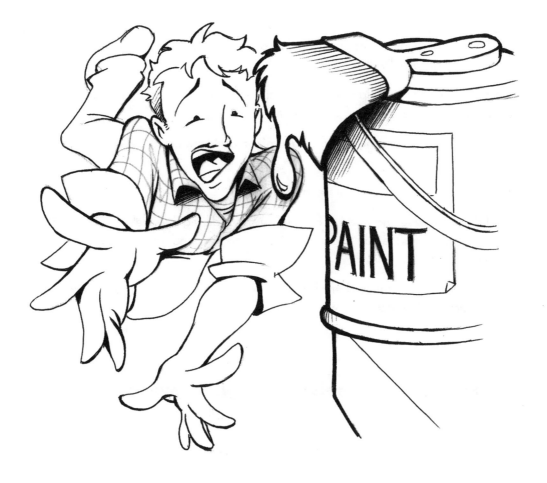

Overcoming Depression
A Five Areas Approach

Section 1 Introduction

This is the second of two workbooks that looks at the area of altered thinking. In this workbook you will:

- briefly review how your **thought investigation** practice went;
- learn how to challenge extreme or unhelpful thoughts;
- develop balanced conclusions and create plans to put them into practice.

Review since the last workbook

In the first workbook in this area *Noticing extreme and unhelpful thinking*, you were asked to try and do several tasks in preparation for this current workbook. **Have you been able to do each of these tasks?** They were to:

- Use the thought investigation worksheet to carry out a thought investigation on **four** occasions when your mood unhelpfully altered.   Yes ☐   No ☐

- **Stop and think** which unhelpful thinking style(s) you noticed during these times and to **reflect** on the helpfulness and accuracy of the thoughts.   Yes ☐   No ☐

- To begin to ask yourself, *are the thoughts actually **true**?* How could I see things more helpfully and accurately – in a less extreme way?   Yes ☐   No ☐

- Q. Have you been able to do each of these tasks?   Yes ☐   No ☐

If yes: Well done. Thinking and working on your problems during the week is an important part of overcoming depression. It is the day-to-day practice of applying what you are learning that will help you to feel better.

If no: This may have been for a number of reasons. Sometimes negative thoughts may act to block carrying out an activity. This workbook will help you begin to learn new skills in how to challenge negative thoughts that can undermine your motivation. Try to use this as an opportunity to change how you think about what you do.

Identifying extreme and unhelpful thoughts: revision

You have already practised identifying extreme and unhelpful thoughts in workbook 4, *Noticing extreme and unhelpful thinking*. In this you learned to:

1 Watch out for times when your mood unhelpfully alters (for example times when you feel more depressed, upset, worried, panicky or angry) and then try to notice what is going through your mind at that time.

2 Use the thought investigation worksheet to record the thoughts that led up to the mood change.

Useful questions to help you identify the immediate thoughts that lead to unhelpfully altered mood can include:

What did I think about:

- myself;

- the current events/situation;

- how others see me;

- what might happen in the future?

- Were there any painful memories from the past?

- Did I notice any images or pictures in my mind?

Thoughts that are **extreme and unhelpful** are the target for change in these workbooks. These are the sort of thoughts that were identified in **columns 4 and 5 of the thought identification worksheet.**

Task from workbook 4

In order to recognise unhelpful and extreme thoughts, in workbook 4 you were asked to identify four times when your mood unhelpfully altered and to complete a thought investigation on each using the **thought investigation worksheet**. In the next section of the workbook, you will learn how to begin to challenge thoughts that are extreme and unhelpful.

Changing extreme and unhelpful thinking

Sometimes people try to cope with depression by **trying not to think about it.** Is this an effective strategy? In order to see how effective it is, try this practical experiment. You will now be asked to try as hard as you can not to think about a common object. Please try very hard for the next 30 seconds **not** to think about a white polar bear.

After you have done this, think about what happened. Was it easy not to think about the white polar bear, or did it take a lot of effort? You may have noticed that trying hard not to think about it actually made it worse and brought thoughts or images of a white polar bear on even more. Alternatively, you may have spent a lot of mental effort trying hard to think about something else such as a black polar bear or something completely different instead.

Conclusion:

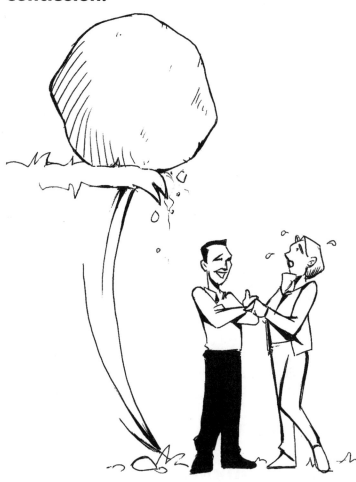

Trying not to think about something can sometimes cause the thought to become **even more** intrusive and troubling. For many people, trying hard to ignore their worries and not think about them is therefore ineffective and may actually worsen the problem. Instead, there is a need to learn new ways of challenging and tackling unhelpful and extreme thoughts.

In depression, it is often the case that the person is not completely fair or accurate in the way they judge themselves and interpret what happens to them. It is rare for someone who is depressed to question the *accuracy* of his or her thoughts. This is important because many negative thoughts are both extreme and inaccurate as well as unhelpful.

You have already learned about **unhelpful thinking styles,** and started to **stop, think and reflect** when you notice these extreme and unhelpful thoughts. The next few pages will introduce you to a step-by-step approach to questioning and challenging these thoughts.

Section 2   Challenging unhelpful thinking styles

The following skills aim to help you to begin to question the stream of extreme and unhelpful thoughts that 'pop' into the mind through the day when someone is depressed. In depression, these unhelpful thinking styles come into mind more often than usual and are more likely to be believed.

Examples of extreme and unhelpful thoughts include:

- *'I'm bad.'*
- *'I messed that up.'*
- *'I'll never get better.'*
- *'It's been a terrible week.'*
- *'Just typical – things **always** go wrong.'*

At the moment it is likely that when you notice thoughts like these you often tend to accept that they are true. You may notice that it is easier to believe such thoughts at times of highly negative emotion such as when you feel very low, anxious or upset.

One effective way to improve how you feel is to practise skills of how to challenge these thoughts. As you become better at this, you will find you are able to challenge the thoughts at more difficult times.

The approach uses a three-point plan to bring about change:

1   **Identify** and rate your belief in the extreme and unhelpful thought(s).
2   **Question** the helpfulness and accuracy of the thought(s).
3   Come to a balanced **conclusion** about the thought(s).

This thought-challenging approach of ***identify, question and conclude*** can help you begin to change the problem of unhelpful and extreme thinking.

You have already practised how to identify and rate extreme thoughts using the **thought investigation worksheet**. This will have helped you to begin to identify one or more thoughts that are present when your mood unhelpfully alters. This process is described in workbook 4 '*Noticing extreme and unhelpful thinking*'.

Revision: Identify an unhelpful thought

Example: Paul's painting

Paul is a 35 year old man who has very high standards. He is currently feeling depressed and has decided to paint his bedroom as a way of increasing his activity levels. He has just completed painting the walls when he realises that a drop of paint has fallen onto the carpet. He immediately feels down and angry with himself.

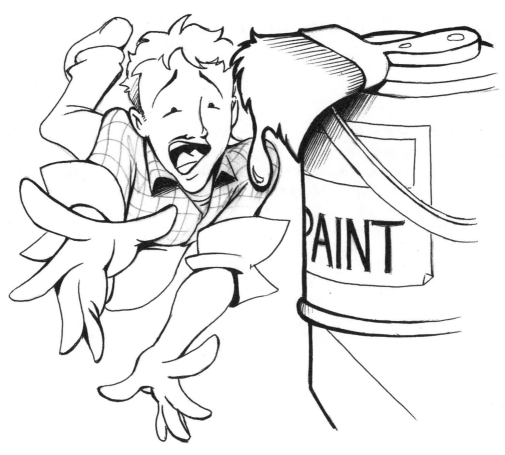

Look at Paul's thought investigation worksheet, where Paul has analysed his reaction to what happened.

Paul's thought investigation worksheet

1 Situation/relationship or practical problem when your mood altered.	2 Altered emotional and physical feelings	3 What immediate thoughts are present at the time?	4 What unhelpful thinking style(s) occur?	5 Impact of the immediate thought(s)
Think in detail: Where am I, what am I doing? Consider: ● **The time**: What time of day is it? ● **The place**: Where am I? ● **The people**: Who is present. Who am I with? ● **The events**: What has been said/What events happened?	Am I ● Low or sad? Guilty? ● Worried, tense, anxious or panicky? ● Angry or irritable? ● Ashamed or suspicious? **a)** State the feelings clearly. Try to be as precise as possible. If more than one feeling occurs, underline the most powerful feeling. **b)** How powerful is this feeling (0–100%)? **c)** Note down any strong physical sensations you notice.	What is going through my mind? How do I see: ● Myself/How others see me? ● The current events/situation. ● What might happen in the future? ● My own body, behaviour or performance? ● Any memories or images? **a)** State the thought(s) clearly. Try to be as precise as possible. If more than one thought occurs, underline the most powerful thought. **b)** Rate how strongly you believe the most powerful thought at the time (0–100%).	1 Bias against myself. 2 Putting a negative slant on things (negative mental filter). 3 Having a gloomy view of the future/ jumping to the worst conclusion. 4 Negative view about how others see me (mind-reading). 5 Bearing all responsibility. 6 Making extreme statements/rules, e.g. using *must*, *should*, *ought*, *always*, and *never* statements. If any of the styles are present, you have identified an **extreme** thought.	**a)** What did I do differently? Consider any: ● Reduced activity. ● Unhelpful behaviours. **b)** What was the impact on: ● Myself? ● My view of others? ● How I felt? ● What I said? ● What I did? ● Overall, was the impact helpful or unhelpful? If there is an unhelpful impact, you have identified an **unhelpful** thought.
Situation: *10 a.m. in the room by myself, painting.* *A drop of paint has fallen on the carpet*	**a) My feelings:** *Down and angry with myself.* **b) Powerfulness:** *0–100% = 90%* **c) Physical sensations:** *Pressure in the pit of my stomach, and a feeling of heaviness in my body.*	**My immediate thought(s):** **a)** ✎ State the thought(s) clearly. *I always mess things up* *The carpet is ruined* If you have noticed more than one thought, **underline** the most powerful thought. **b)** Rate your belief in the most powerful thought at the time: 0% ⎸————————⎹ 100% ——×——	**Which thinking styles are present?** (please state numbers or types) ✎ No(s): *1, 2, 6* *for most of the next week*	**a) What did I do differently?** *I went to bed and avoided doing tasks where things can go wrong* **b)** Overall, is it **helpful** or **unhelpful** for me to believe the thought? Helpful ☐ Unhelpful ✓

For this example, Paul believed the thought '*I always mess things up*' **75 per cent of the time.** This is the most powerful thought that he noticed going through his mind at the time his mood unhelpfully altered. The fact that believing the thought shows one of the unhelpful thinking styles and is unhelpful for Paul is an important thing for Paul to have noticed. If it is unhelpful, then why focus his time and energy on thinking it? Can Paul change from this unhelpful focus to a more **helpful focus** to his thinking?

You will now see how Paul goes through the process of coming to a more balanced and helpful way of seeing things.

Questioning unhelpful thoughts

---

i   Is the thought actually true?

Q. What is the evidence <u>for</u> and <u>against</u> the immediate thought?

Evidence <u>supporting</u> the immediate extreme thought

First, Paul is asked to think about **why** he believes the negative thought.

Paul's answer:
*Well, when I did the painting, a drip **did** fall onto the carpet. It was only a small drip, but it was there. If you looked, you could see it. I guess that maybe that isn't really enough to say that I messed **everything** up.*

Q. Can you show that the thought is correct from what you know to be true?

Yes ☐   No ✔

Evidence <u>against</u> the immediate extreme thought:

Q. Is there anything to make you think the thought is incorrect?   Yes ✔   No ☐

Paul's answer:
I had been painting for hours and was tired. I had put down dustsheets and they caught most of the drips. The rest of the painting went well. I even saw the drip so that I could clean it up and avoiding trampling it all over the house. I can't be expected to get everything right. It's silly to say 'I always mess things up' – it was just one drip.

Q. Are there any other ways of explaining the situation that are more accurate?   Yes ✔   No ☐

Paul's answer:
I actually did a good job. I prepared for it well, and the end job looks good. I should give myself credit for the positive job I did rather than focusing on one small thing that went wrong.

---

ii   Q. If I wasn't feeling like this, would I believe the thought?

Yes ☐   No ✔

Paul's answer:
It must be the depression. Normally I would have just tried to clean up the drip or move some furniture to cover it up. I would have said 'so what' and got on with things. The depression must be affecting how I feel.

---

iii   Do I apply one set of standards to myself and another to others?

Q. Are the standards that you set yourself higher than those you expect others to achieve?

Yes ✔   No ☐

Paul's answer:
Definitely. I've always been like that.

Q. Would you tell a friend who believed the same thought that they were wrong?

Yes ✔   No ☐

Paul's answer:
I'd tell them, 'What are you saying – you're just being silly. The rest of the painting went well and the room looks great. Stop criticising yourself like that. You're just focusing on the drop of paint rather than the whole picture. You managed to use turps to remove most of the mark and it hasn't spoiled the floor. You don't <u>always</u> mess everything up.' I'd also say, 'Look at all the other things you have done this week. Give yourself due credit'.

iv   Change your perspective: What would other people say?

Q. Have you heard *different opinions* from others about the thought you hold?   Yes ✔   No ☐

Paul's answer:
Other people have said it looks good. My friend Anne liked it and I trust her to say what she really thinks. Maybe I am wrong to say 'I always mess things up'. Anne doesn't think that.

Come to a balanced conclusion

Use the answers to the previous questions to come up with a balanced and helpful conclusion. Try to be honest with yourself. A *balanced conclusion* is based on **all** the information you have available to you at the time.

Paul's conclusion:

'The painting didn't go completely right, but I've managed to clean up the small spot of paint that I dropped. There is a mark there, but its hardly noticeable. The rest of the room looks good and I'm a good painter. I have also got some other things right this week. I need to be less harsh on myself.'

Re-rate your belief in the *immediate extreme thought* and the *new balanced conclusion*.

Summary: In Paul's example:

Immediate thought: *'I always mess things up'*

a) Paul's belief in the immediate thought **at the time he had it**.

0 per cent _____×_____ 100 per cent
Don't believe at all   Believe fully

b) Paul's belief in the immediate thought **now**:

0 per cent _____×_____ 100 per cent
Don't believe at all   Believe fully

After challenging the belief, the thought is now believed only **25 per cent**.

Balanced conclusion: *'The painting didn't go completely right, but I've managed to clean up the small spot of paint that I dropped. There is a mark there, but its hardly noticeable. The rest of the room looks good and I'm a good painter. I have also got some other things right this week. I need to be less harsh on myself.'*

Paul's belief in the balanced conclusion:

0 per cent _____×_____ 100 per cent
Don't believe at all   Believe fully

Summary

- Paul now believes the **immediate thought only 25 per cent** (compared to 75 per cent before).
- Paul believes the new **balanced conclusion 90 per cent.**

Paul has successfully challenged his original extreme and unhelpful thought. This process can be repeated for any other extreme and unhelpful thoughts.

An important thing for Paul to do, is to begin to make changes in his life so that he can act to reinforce the balanced conclusion, and to undermine the original extreme thought that '*I always mess things up*'.

Putting the balanced conclusion into practice

One helpful approach to find out whether the new balanced conclusion is true and helpful is to **set up a test** to see if it is true in practice. What test(s) could Paul set up? For example, Paul could ask other friends what they really think about the painting and how the room looks in order to obtain someone else's opinion on the matter.

One powerful action you can do to test the helpfulness and accuracy of the balanced conclusion is to **act on the balanced conclusion,** believing it to be true, and see what happens. This may mean choosing to do the **reverse** of what the immediate thought may be telling you.

Example: You are asked to a party. Your initial reaction is to say no as a result of an immediate thought '*I won't enjoy it*'. Try to act against this thought (by going to the party) in order to test out whether it is true. You may well find that the party goes better than you predicted and that you do enjoy it at least a little.

Important point: By far the best evidence for or against a thought is found through looking at the consequences of what happens when you choose to act or not act on it. **Reinforce** your balanced conclusions by acting on them. **Undermine** your negative thoughts by acting against them.

Paul's plan for putting the balanced conclusion into practice

1   *I am going to choose to have a **more helpful focus for my thinking**: I'm going to set aside some time to think back on those things where I have a sense of achievement. I am going to choose to look at the whole room that I've painted, and not unhelpfully focus on the small spot of paint that is hardly noticeable.*

2   *I am going to choose to keep doing the painting and I am going to do this at a sensible pace. I will do the skirting boards tomorrow. That will help me to **undermine** that old thought that I always mess things up because it will mean me **acting against** my tendency to go to bed and stop doing things. Sure, some things won't go completely right, but lots of things will go well, and it will be a lot more helpful for me to focus on these. Anyway, who does get everything right?*

3   *I'm going to ask my other friends what they think of the room and see if they mention the spot of paint on the carpet. Now I come to think of it, I bet they don't (and in fact when he asks two other friends, they don't mention it at all. They do however say how impressed they are with the room).*

   Q. Have you created a **plan** to put the balanced conclusion into practice?   Yes ✔   No ☐

The impact of balanced thoughts

The purpose of showing you this example is to try to illustrate the process of challenging unhelpful and extreme thoughts. By asking the series of questions, Paul was able to begin to produce an alternative conclusion that is:

1 helpful;

2 more balanced and true.

You will now have the opportunity to practise these skills for yourself on one of your own unhelpful and extreme thoughts.

Section 3 Practice: challenging your own unhelpful thoughts

Identifying an unhelpful thought

Identify a negative, extreme or unhelpful thought

It is best at first to choose a thought that is an extreme and unhelpful reaction to something that has happened or that has been said.

● Choose just one thought to question at a time.

● Clearly identify and write down what the thought is.

● For the time being avoid thoughts such as *'I am ...'*, *'People are ...'*, *'the World is ...'* because these sorts of thoughts are often very difficult to challenge at first.

Use your **thought investigation worksheet** or recent experiences to identify a thought.

✎ Write any immediate thoughts you noticed here:

```
┌────────────────────────────────────────────┐
│                                              │
│                                              │
│                                              │
│                                              │
│                                              │
└────────────────────────────────────────────┘
```

Assessing my <u>belief</u> in the most powerful extreme and negative immediate thought

Choose the thought that seemed to have the greatest emotional impact on you:

✎ Write it here:

```
┌────────────────────────────────────────────┐
│                                              │
│                                              │
│                                              │
└────────────────────────────────────────────┘
```

Rate how much did you believe the most powerful thought at that time.

Make a cross on the line below to record how much you believed the thought.

Not at all _____ Completely believed
       0 per cent   50 per cent   100 per cent

The following are a series of questions that you should consider in order to challenge and test out whether this extreme thought is either helpful or true. As you answer these questions, please try to **stop, think and reflect** as this is an important part of the process of change.

Questioning unhelpful thoughts

Is the thought actually true?

---

i   **Q. What is the evidence for and against the immediate thought?**

Evidence supporting the immediate thought:

First, think about **why** you believe the negative thought.

✎ Write this down here:

My reasons:

```



```

Can you show that the thought is correct from what you know to be true?   Yes ☐   No ☐

Evidence *against* the immediate thought:

Q. Is there anything to make you think the thought is incorrect?   Yes ☐   No ☐

✎ **My comments**:

```



```

Q. Are there any other ways of explaining the situation that are more accurate?   Yes ☐   No ☐

✎ **My comments**:

```



```

---

ii   Q. If I wasn't feeling like this, would I believe the thought?   Yes ☐   No ☐
✎ **My comments**:

iii   Do I apply one set of standards to myself and another to others?

Q. Are the standards that you set yourself higher than those you expect others to achieve?

Yes ☐   No ☐

✎ **My comments**:

Q. Would you tell a friend who believed the same thought that they were wrong?   Yes ☐   No ☐

✎ **My comments**:

iv   Change your perspective: What would other people say?

Q. Have you heard *different opinions* from others about the thought you hold?   Yes ☐   No ☐

✎ **My comments**:

Come to a balanced conclusion

Use the answers to the previous questions to come up with a balanced conclusion. Try to be honest with yourself. A *balanced conclusion* is based on **all** the information you have available to you at the time.

My balanced conclusion

✎ Please write your new balanced conclusion into the space below:

Summary

Re-rate your belief in the immediate extreme thought and the new balanced conclusion

My immediate extreme thought:

✎ *Write here:*

My belief in the immediate thought **at the time I had it**:

(Make a cross on the line below to record how much you believed the thought)

0 per cent ————————————————————— **100 per cent**
Don't believe at all   Believe fully

My belief in the immediate thought **now**:

0 per cent ————————————————————— **100 per cent**
Don't believe at all   Believe fully

My balanced conclusion:

✎ *Write in your balanced conclusion here:*

My belief in my new balanced conclusion:

(Make a cross on the line below to record how much you believe the thought)

0 per cent ————————————————————— **100 per cent**
Don't believe at all   Believe fully

The series of questions that you have answered have helped you to **stop, think and reflect** on your immediate thought in a structured way. Look at the rating of the amount you believe the immediate thought **before and after** this questioning process. If the amount you believe the immediate extreme belief has dropped, this is a sign that you have been able (at least in part) to challenge the immediate thought. If this proved difficult, don't give up. It takes time to learn skills of effectively questioning and challenging unhelpful thoughts. It may be difficult at first to break the habit of extreme and negative thinking particularly if you have been depressed for some time. Keep trying though, and you will find that it becomes easier.

One important way of reducing the strength of your unhelpful and extreme thoughts is to **act against them** and **put your balanced conclusion into practice.**

Putting your balanced conclusion into practice

One helpful approach to find out whether your new balanced conclusion is true and helpful is to **set up a test** to see if it is true in practice. By far the best evidence for or against a thought is found through looking at the consequences of what happens when you choose to act or not act on it. **Reinforce** your balanced conclusions by acting on them. **Undermine** your negative thoughts by acting against them. Try to create a **plan** to do this.

Please write into the workbook your own plan to **undermine** the immediate thought, or to **reinforce** the new balanced conclusion.

My plan for putting my balanced conclusion into practice

To undermine the immediate thought:

To reinforce my new balanced conclusion:

Have you created a **plan** to put your balanced conclusion into practice?   Yes ☐   No ☐

If yes, put this into practice and discuss what you learn with your health care practitioner. If you have not been able to think up a plan, discuss this with your health care practitioner who will help you think how you may be able to re-inforce your balanced conclusion and put it into practice.

The questions you have worked through can be applied to any extreme and unhelpful thoughts that result in an unhelpfully altered mood. By examining, questioning and challenging these thoughts, you will begin to change the way you see yourself, your current situation and the future.

KEY POINTS
- Begin to pay attention to and to challenge any unhelpful and extreme thoughts.
- Your negative, extreme and unhelpful thoughts will slowly change as you begin to challenge them in a regular way. By continuing to do this, you will develop more balanced, moderate and helpful thinking.

In order to help you practise the skills of questioning and challenging unhelpful thoughts, a **thought challenge worksheet** has been developed. Together with the thought investigation worksheet you used in workbook 4, the two sides of the Worksheet allow you to identify and then challenge unhelpful and extreme thoughts.

● Side 1 is the *thought investigation worksheet* you used in the previous workbook to help you to identify extreme and unhelpful thoughts.

● Side 2 is the *thought challenge worksheet*. This consists of questions to help you complete the thought challenge process that you have practiced in the current workbook.

You will find copies of the worksheet at the end of the workbook. You can tear these out or photocopy them if you wish. Try to carry them around with you in order to help you to identify and challenge any unhelpful and extreme thoughts. With practice, you will find that it becomes easier to do this and you will be able to develop more balanced, moderate and helpful thinking.

Section 4 **Workbook summary**

In this workbook you have:

● briefly reviewed how your **thought investigation** practice went;

● learned and practised how to challenge extreme or unhelpful thoughts;

● developed balanced conclusions and created plans to put them into practice.

Putting into practice what you have learned

You have already begun to identify important changes in what you think and do. To build on this please can you:

> Use the two sides of the **thought worksheet** to help you go through the process of **identifying, questioning and challenging** extreme and unhelpful thoughts on **four** occasions when your mood alters during the next week.

If you have difficulties with this, don't worry. Just do what you can and discuss any problems with your health care practitioner.

Once you have completed four worksheets over the next week, it is advisable to continue practising this approach using the worksheets over a number of weeks. With practice you will find that you become skilled at using this approach, and can begin to identify and challenge extreme thoughts without the help of the worksheet. You will find copies of the **thought worksheet** at the back of the workbook.

My notes

....
....
....
....
....
....
....
....
....
....
....
....
....
....
....
....
....
....
....
....
....
....
....
....

My notes ....
....

Practice 1   Thought investigation worksheet (side 1): identifying extreme and unhelpful thinking

1 Situation/relationship or practical problem when your mood altered.	2 Altered emotional and physical feelings	3 What immediate thoughts are present at the time?	4 What unhelpful thinking style(s) occur?	5 Impact of the immediate thought(s)
Think in detail: Where am I, what am I doing? Consider: ●**The time**: What time of day is it? ●**The place**: Where am I? ●**The people**: Who is present? Who am I with? ●**The events**: What has been said/What events happened?	Am I ● Low or sad? Guilty? ● Worried, tense, anxious or panicky? ● Angry or irritable? ● Ashamed or suspicious? **a)** State the feelings clearly. Try to be as precise as possible. If more than one feeling occurs, underline the most powerful feeling. **b)** How powerful is this feeling (0–100%)? **c)** Note down any strong physical sensations you notice.	What is going through my mind? How do I see: ● Myself, How others see me? ● The current events/situation. ● What might happen in the future? ● My own body, behaviour or performance? ● Any memories or images? **a)** State the thought(s) clearly. Try to be as precise as possible. If more than one thought occurs, underline the most powerful thought. **b)** Rate how strongly you believe the most powerful thought at the time (0–100%).	1 Bias against myself. 2 Putting a negative slant on things (negative mental filter). 3 Having a gloomy view of the future/ jumping to the worst conclusion. 4 Negative view about how others see me (mind-reading). 5 Bearing all responsibility. 6 Making extreme statements/rules, e.g. using *must, should, ought, always,* and *never statements.* If any of the styles are present, you have identified an **extreme** thought.	**a)** What did I do differently? Consider any: ● Reduced activity. ● Unhelpful behaviours. **b)** What was the impact on: ● Myself? ● My view of others? ● How I felt? ● What I said? ● What I did? ● Overall, was the impact helpful or unhelpful? If there is an unhelpful impact, you have identified an **unhelpful** thought.
Situation:	**a) My feelings:** **b) Powerfulness:** 0–100% = **c) Physical sensations:**	**My immediate thought(s):** **a)** ✐ State the thought(s) clearly. If you have noticed more than one thought, **underline** the most powerful thought. **b)** ✐ Rate your belief in the most powerful thought at the time: 0% 100%	**Which thinking styles are present?** (please state numbers or types) ✐ No(s):	**a)** What did I do differently? **b)** Overall, is it **helpful** or **unhelpful** for me to believe the thought? Helpful ☐ Unhelpful ☐

Thought challenge worksheet (side 2): choose one thought to challenge at a time

6 Reasons supporting the immediate thought	7 Evidence against the immediate thought	8 Come to a balanced conclusion	9 My plan for putting the balanced conclusion into practice
List all the reasons why I believed the immediate thought at the time.	☐ Is there anything to make me think the thought is incorrect? ☐ Are there any other ways of explaining the situation that are more accurate? ☐ If I wasn't feeling depressed, what would I say? ☐ Would I tell a friend who believed the same thought that they were wrong? What would other people say? ☐ Have I heard *different* opinions from others about the thought?	Use the answers from columns 6 and 7 to try to come up with a **balanced** and **helpful** conclusion. Look for a *balanced conclusion* that you can believe. This should be based on **all** the information you have available to you and bear in mind the reasons for and against believing the immediate thought.	● How can I change what I do to reinforce my balanced conclusion? ● How can I undermine my immediate negative thought by acting against it?
My evidence supporting the immediate thought: (write in)	**My evidence against the immediate thought**: (write in)	**My balanced conclusion**: (write in) **a)** Rating of my belief in the balanced conclusion: 0% 100% **b)** Re-rate my belief in the immediate thought: 0% 100%	**My plan** to put the balanced conclusion into practice: (write in)

Practice 2 Thought investigation worksheet (side 1): identifying extreme and unhelpful thinking

1 Situation/relationship or practical problem when your mood altered.	2 Altered emotional and physical feelings	3 What immediate thoughts are present at the time?	4 What unhelpful thinking style(s) occur?	5 Impact of the immediate thought(s)
Think in detail: Where am I, what am I doing? Consider: • **The time**: What time of day is it? • **The place**: Where am I? • **The people**: Who is present? Who am I with? • **The events**: What has been said/What events happened?	Am I • Low or sad? Guilty? • Worried, tense, anxious or panicky? • Angry or irritable? • Ashamed or suspicious? **a)** State the feelings clearly. Try to be as precise as possible. If more than one feeling occurs, underline the most powerful feeling. **b)** How powerful is this feeling (0–100%)? **c)** Note down any strong physical sensations you notice.	What is going through my mind? How do I see: • Myself, How others see me? • The current events/situation. • What might happen in the future? • My own body, behaviour or performance? • Any memories or images? **a)** State the thought(s) clearly. Try to be as precise as possible. If more than one thought occurs, underline the most powerful thought. **b)** Rate how strongly you believe the most powerful thought at the time (0–100%).	1 Bias against myself. 2 Putting a negative slant on things (negative mental filter). 3 Having a gloomy view of the future/ jumping to the worst conclusion. 4 Negative view about how others see me (mind-reading). 5 Bearing all responsibility. 6 Making extreme statements/rules, e.g. using *must, should, ought, always,* and *never* statements. If any of the styles are present, you have identified an **extreme** thought.	**a)** What did I do differently? Consider any: • Reduced activity. • Unhelpful behaviours. **b)** What was the impact on: • Myself? • My view of others? • How I felt? • What I said? • What I did? • Overall, was the impact helpful or unhelpful? If there is an unhelpful impact, you have identified an **unhelpful** thought.
Situation:	**a) My feelings:** **b) Powerfulness:** 0–100% = **c) Physical sensations:**	**My immediate thought(s):** **a)** ✐ State the thought(s) clearly. If you have noticed more than one thought, **underline** the most powerful thought. **b)** ✐ Rate your belief in the most powerful thought at the time 0%　　　　　　100%	**Which thinking styles are present?** (please state numbers or types) ✐ No(s):	**a)** What did I do differently? **b)** Overall, is it **helpful** or **unhelpful** for me to believe the thought? Helpful ☐ Unhelpful ☐

Thought challenge worksheet (side 2): choose one thought to challenge at a time

6 Reasons supporting the immediate thought	7 Evidence against the immediate thought	8 Come to a balanced conclusion	9 My plan for putting the balanced conclusion into practice
List all the reasons why I believed the immediate thought at the time.	☐ Is there anything to make me think the thought is incorrect? ☐ Are there any other ways of explaining the situation that are more accurate? ☐ If I wasn't feeling depressed, what would I say? ☐ Would I tell a friend who believed the same thought that they were wrong? What would other people say? ☐ Have I heard *different opinions* from others about the thought?	Use the answers from columns 6 and 7 to try to come up with a **balanced** and **helpful** conclusion. Look for a *balanced conclusion* that you can believe. This should be based on **all** the information you have available to you and bear in mind the reasons for and against believing the immediate thought.	● How can I change what I do to reinforce my balanced conclusion? ● How can I undermine my immediate negative thought by acting against it?
My evidence supporting the immediate thought: (write in)	**My evidence against the immediate thought:** (write in)	**My balanced conclusion:** (write in) **a)** Rating of my belief in the balanced conclusion: 0% 100% **b)** Re-rate my belief in the immediate thought: 0% 100%	**My plan** to put the balanced conclusion into practice: (write in)

Practice 3   Thought investigation worksheet (side 1): identifying extreme and unhelpful thinking

1 Situation/relationship or practical problem when your mood altered.	2 Altered emotional and physical feelings	3 What immediate thoughts are present at the time?	4 What unhelpful thinking style(s) occur?	5 Impact of the immediate thought(s)
Think in detail: Where am I, what am I doing? Consider: ● **The time**: What time of day is it? ● **The place**: Where am I? ● **The people**: Who is present? Who am I with? ● **The events**: What has been said/What events happened?	Am I ● Low or sad? Guilty? ● Worried, tense, anxious or panicky? ● Angry or irritable? ● Ashamed or suspicious? **a)** State the feelings clearly. Try to be as precise as possible. If more than one feeling occurs, underline the most powerful feeling. **b)** How powerful is this feeling (0–100%)? **c)** Note down any strong physical sensations you notice.	What is going through my mind? How do I see: ● Myself, How others see me? ● The current events/situation. ● What might happen in the future? ● My own body, behaviour or performance? ● Any memories or images? **a)** State the thought(s) clearly. Try to be as precise as possible. If more than one thought occurs, underline the most powerful thought. **b)** Rate how strongly you believe the most powerful thought at the time (0–100%).	1 Bias against myself. 2 Putting a negative slant on things (negative mental filter). 3 Having a gloomy view of the future/ jumping to the worst conclusion. 4 Negative view about how others see me (mind-reading). 5 Bearing all responsibility. 6 Making extreme statements/rules, e.g. using *must, should, ought, always,* and *never* statements. If any of the styles are present, you have identified an **extreme** thought.	**a)** What did I do differently? Consider any: ● Reduced activity. ● Unhelpful behaviours. **b)** What was the impact on: ● Myself? ● My view of others? ● How I felt? ● What I said? ● What I did? ● Overall, was the impact helpful or unhelpful? If there is an unhelpful impact, you have identified an **unhelpful** thought.
Situation:	**a) My feelings:** **b) Powerfulness:** 0–100% = **c) Physical sensations:**	**My immediate thought(s):** **a)** ✐ State the thought(s) clearly. If you have noticed more than one thought, **underline** the most powerful thought. **b)** ✐ Rate your belief in the most powerful thought at the time: 0% 100%	**Which thinking styles are present?** (please state numbers or types) ✐ No(s):	**a)** What did I do differently? **b)** Overall, is it **helpful** or **unhelpful** for me to believe the thought? Helpful ☐ Unhelpful ☐

Thought challenge worksheet (side 2): choose one thought to challenge at a time

6 Reasons supporting the immediate thought	7 Evidence against the immediate thought	8 Come to a balanced conclusion	9 My plan for putting the balanced conclusion into practice
List all the reasons why I believed the immediate thought at the time.	☐ Is there anything to make me think the thought is incorrect? ☐ Are there any other ways of explaining the situation that are more accurate? ☐ If I wasn't feeling depressed, what would I say? ☐ Would I tell a friend who believed the same thought that they were wrong? What would other people say? ☐ Have I heard *different opinions* from others about the thought?	Use the answers from columns 6 and 7 to try to come up with a **balanced** and **helpful** conclusion. Look for a *balanced conclusion* that you can believe. This should be based on **all** the information you have available to you and bear in mind the reasons for and against believing the immediate thought.	● How can I change what I do to reinforce my balanced conclusion? ● How can I undermine my immediate negative thought by acting against it?
My evidence supporting the immediate thought: (write in)	**My evidence against the immediate thought:** (write in)	**My balanced conclusion:** (write in) **a)** Rating of my belief in the balanced conclusion: 0% 100% **b)** Re-rate my belief in the immediate thought: 0% 100%	**My plan** to put the balanced conclusion into practice: (write in)

Practice 4   Thought investigation worksheet (side 1): identifying extreme and unhelpful thinking

1 Situation/relationship or practical problem when your mood altered.	2 Altered emotional and physical feelings	3 What immediate thoughts are present at the time?	4 What unhelpful thinking style(s) occur?	5 Impact of the immediate thought(s)
Think in detail: Where am I, what am I doing? Consider: • **The time**: What time of day is it? • **The place**: Where am I? • **The people**: Who is present? Who am I with? • **The events**: What has been said/What events happened?	Am I • Low or sad? Guilty? • Worried, tense, anxious or panicky? • Angry or irritable? • Ashamed or suspicious? **a)** State the feelings clearly. Try to be as precise as possible. If more than one feeling occurs, underline the most powerful feeling. **b)** How powerful is this feeling (0–100%)? **c)** Note down any strong physical sensations you notice.	What is going through my mind? How do I see: • Myself, How others see me? • The current events/situation. • What might happen in the future? • My own body, behaviour or performance? • Any memories or images? **a)** State the thought(s) clearly. Try to be as precise as possible. If more than one thought occurs, underline the most powerful thought. **b)** Rate how strongly you believe the most powerful thought at the time (0–100%).	1 Bias against myself. 2 Putting a negative slant on things (negative mental filter). 3 Having a gloomy view of the future/jumping to the worst conclusion. 4 Negative view about how others see me (mind-reading). 5 Bearing all responsibility. 6 Making extreme statements/rules, e.g. using *must, should, ought, always,* and *never* statements. If any of the styles are present, you have identified an **extreme** thought.	**a)** What did I do differently? Consider any: • Reduced activity. • Unhelpful behaviours. **b)** What was the impact on: • Myself? • My view of others? • How I felt? • What I said? • What I did? • Overall, was the impact helpful or unhelpful? If there is an unhelpful impact, you have identified an **unhelpful** thought.
Situation:	**a) My feelings:** **b) Powerfulness:** 0–100% = **c) Physical sensations:**	**My immediate thought(s):** **a)** ✎ State the thought(s) clearly. If you have noticed more than one thought, **underline** the most powerful thought. **b)** ✎ Rate your belief in the most powerful thought at the time: 0% 100%	**Which thinking styles are present?** (please state numbers or types) ✎ No(s):	**a)** What did I do differently? **b)** Overall, is it **helpful** or **unhelpful** for me to believe the thought? Helpful ☐ Unhelpful ☐

Thought challenge worksheet (side 2): choose one thought to challenge at a time

6 Reasons supporting the immediate thought	7 Evidence against the immediate thought	8 Come to a balanced conclusion	9 My plan for putting the balanced conclusion into practice
List all the reasons why I believed the immediate thought at the time.	☐ Is there anything to make me think the thought is incorrect? ☐ Are there any other ways of explaining the situation that are more accurate? ☐ If I wasn't feeling depressed, what would I say? ☐ Would I tell a friend who believed the same thought that they were wrong? What would other people say? ☐ Have I heard *different opinions* from others about the thought?	Use the answers from columns 6 and 7 to try to come up with a **balanced** and **helpful** conclusion. Look for a *balanced conclusion* that you can believe. This should be based on **all** the information you have available to you and bear in mind the reasons for and against believing the immediate thought.	● How can I change what I do to reinforce my balanced conclusion? ● How can I undermine my immediate negative thought by acting against it?
My evidence supporting the immediate thought: (write in)	**My evidence against the immediate thought:** (write in)	**My balanced conclusion:** (write in) **a)** Rating of my belief in the balanced conclusion: 0% 100% **b)** Re-rate my belief in the immediate thought: 0% 100%	**My plan** to put the balanced conclusion into practice: (write in)

Thought investigation worksheet (side 1): identifying extreme and unhelpful thinking

1 Situation/relationship or practical problem when your mood altered.	2 Altered emotional and physical feelings	3 What immediate thoughts are present at the time?	4 What unhelpful thinking style(s) occur?	5 Impact of the immediate thought(s)
Think in detail: Where am I, what am I doing? Consider: ●**The time**: What time of day is it? ●**The place**: Where am I? ●**The people**: Who is present? Who am I with? ●**The events**: What has been said/What events happened?	Am I ● Low or sad? Guilty? ● Worried, tense, anxious or panicky? ● Angry or irritable? ● Ashamed or suspicious? **a)** State the feelings clearly. Try to be as precise as possible. If more than one feeling occurs, underline the most powerful feeling. **b)** How powerful is this feeling (0–100%)? **c)** Note down any strong physical sensations you notice.	What is going through my mind? How do I see: ● Myself, How others see me? ● The current events/situation. ● What might happen in the future? ● My own body, behaviour or performance? ● Any memories or images? **a)** State the thought(s) clearly. Try to be as precise as possible. If more than one thought occurs, underline the most powerful thought. **b)** Rate how strongly you believe the most powerful thought at the time (0–100%).	1 Bias against myself. 2 Putting a negative slant on things (negative mental filter). 3 Having a gloomy view of the future/jumping to the worst conclusion. 4 Negative view about how others see me (mind-reading). 5 Bearing all responsibility. 6 Making extreme statements/rules, e.g. using *must, should, ought, always,* and *never* statements. If any of the styles are present, you have identified an **extreme** thought.	**a)** What did I do differently? Consider any: ● Reduced activity. ● Unhelpful behaviours. **b)** What was the impact on: ● Myself? ● My view of others? ● How I felt? ● What I said? ● What I did? ● Overall, was the impact helpful or unhelpful? If there is an unhelpful impact, you have identified an **unhelpful** thought.
Situation:	**a) My feelings:** **b) Powerfulness:** 0–100% = **c) Physical sensations:**	**My immediate thought(s):** **a)** ✐ State the thought(s) clearly. If you have noticed more than one thought, underline the most powerful thought. **b)** ✐ Rate your belief in the most powerful thought at the time: 0% 100%	**Which thinking styles are present?** (please state numbers or types) ✐ No(s):	**a)** What did I do differently? **b)** Overall, is it **helpful** or **unhelpful** for me to believe the thought? Helpful ☐ Unhelpful ☐

Thought challenge worksheet (side 2): choose one thought to challenge at a time

6 Reasons supporting the immediate thought	7 Evidence against the immediate thought	8 Come to a balanced conclusion	9 My plan for putting the balanced conclusion into practice
List all the reasons why I believed the immediate thought at the time.	☐ Is there anything to make me think the thought is incorrect? ☐ Are there any other ways of explaining the situation that are more accurate? ☐ If I wasn't feeling depressed, what would I say? ☐ Would I tell a friend who believed the same thought that they were wrong? What would other people say? ☐ Have I heard *different opinions* from others about the thought?	Use the answers from columns 6 and 7 to try to come up with a **balanced** and **helpful** conclusion. Look for a *balanced conclusion* that you can believe. This should be based on **all** the information you have available to you and bear in mind the reasons for and against believing the immediate thought.	● How can I change what I do to reinforce my balanced conclusion? ● How can I undermine my immediate negative thought by acting against it?
My evidence supporting the immediate thought: (write in)	**My evidence against the immediate thought:** (write in)	**My balanced conclusion:** (write in) **a)** Rating of my belief in the balanced conclusion: 0% 100% **b)** Re-rate my belief in the immediate thought: 0% 100%	**My plan** to put the balanced conclusion into practice: (write in)

Workbook 6
Changing altered behaviours: reduced activity

Dr Chris Williams

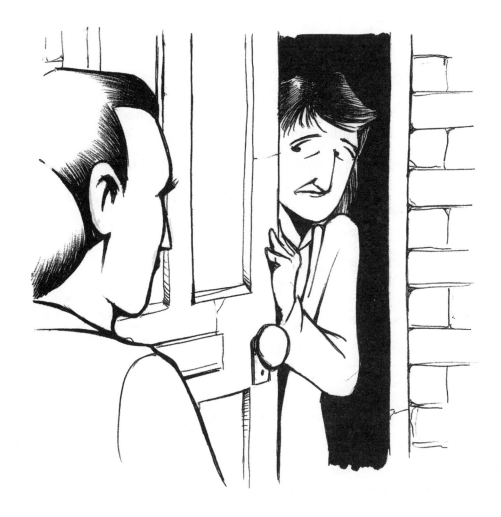

Overcoming Depression
A Five Areas Approach

Section 1   **Introduction**

In this workbook you will:
- revise the vicious circle of reduced activity;
- see an example of a person called Muriel who plans a way of increasing her activity levels;
- practise this approach yourself and review how your planned activity went;
- plan a further activity to put into practice.

In workbook 1 (*Understanding depression*), you looked at how depression may result in:
- A *vicious circle of reduced activity*: stopping doing things that previously gave you a sense of pleasure or achievement. For example you may have stopped reading, or going out, or meeting up with friends or doing hobbies. By removing these things your depression worsens as a result. These changes will be targets for change within the current workbook.
- A *vicious circle of unhelpful behaviours*: starting (or increasing) behaviours that might act to worsen your depression and keep you depressed. This might include starting drinking, becoming very dependent on others, trying to spend your way out of depression, etc. You will find out about this within workbook 7.

When you become depressed, it is normal to find it is difficult doing things. This is because of:
- low energy and tiredness ('*I'm too tired*');
- low mood and little sense of enjoyment or achievement when things are done;
- negative thinking and reduced enthusiasm to do things ('*I just can't be bothered*').

It can sometimes feel as though **everything is too much effort. A vicious circle of reduced activity** may result.

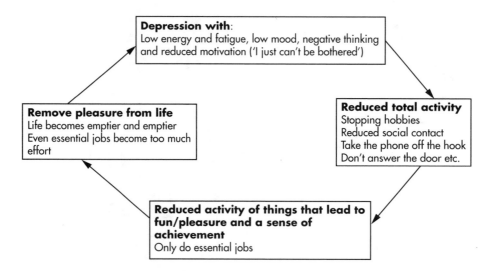

Figure 6.1 The vicious circle of reduced activity

If this vicious circle is happening to you, this workbook will help you to make changes in what you do. To break this vicious circle, you will need a clear plan involving a number of steps in order to bring about lasting change.

Choosing targets for change

You may have tried all sorts of previous attempts to change, but unless you have a clear plan and stick to it, change will be difficult. Planning and selecting which behaviours to try and change first is a crucial part of successfully moving forwards. By choosing which activities to focus on to start with, this also means that you are actively choosing at first **not** to focus on other areas.

Setting **targets** will help you to focus on how to make the changes needed to get better. To do this you will need:

- **short-term** targets: thinking about changes you can make today, tomorrow and the next week;

- **medium-term** targets: changes to be put in place over the next few weeks;

- **long-term targets**: where you want to be in 6 months or a year.

Think about and answer for yourself these questions:

Q. What might be the advantage of planning to change just one reduced activity at first?

Write your answer here:

Q. What are the potential dangers of trying to change *everything* at once?

Write your answer here:

Section 2   Overcoming reduced activity

By working through the seven steps outlined below you can learn an approach that will help you to plan clear ways of overcoming your reduced activity.

Example: Problems of reduced activity

Muriel is a 55 year old woman who has had depression for 3 months. She lives alone and since becoming depressed, she has slowly withdrawn from going out, and has asked her sister Mary to stop visiting her. Her short-term targets are to feel better and 'To do more'.

Compare her plan 'to do more' against the questions for effective change:

The questions for effective change:

1 Will it be useful for understanding or changing how she is?   Yes ☐   No ☐

2 Is it a **specific task** so that she will know when she has done it?   Yes ☐   No ☐

3 Is it **realistic**: is it practical and achievable for her?   Yes ☐   No ☐

4 Does it make clear **what** she is going to do and **when** she is going to do it? Yes ☐   No ☐

5 Is it an activity that won't be easily blocked or prevented by practical problems? Yes ☐   No ☐

Although her goal at first sight sounds to be good, it is **not specific** enough. It does not tell her **what** to do nor defines the steps needed to reach the goal. Because of this, her plan fails the *questions for effective change* test. Poorly defined activities do not address the questions '**What am I going to do?**' and '**When am I going to do it?**' and Muriel's goals therefore need to be changed in order to help her have a clearer plan of what to do. The danger is that she will fail to make useful changes if she uses this current plan, and this may worsen how she feels.

Muriel's first task then is to decide on a specific action that she can do to help overcome her general problem of reduced activity. A **specific** reduced activity she has noticed is that she has stopped meeting people.

Step 1: Clearly define the reduced activity that needs to be changed. Be as precise as possible

---

Muriel's problem area:

*I've identified lots of things on my five areas assessment list. I think the problem I am going to focus on is that **I need to start meeting up with people again**. I've really stopped doing things lately. I'll put the other areas like getting rid of my negative thinking on one side for the moment.*

Q. Is this a clear, focused activity?   Yes ✓   No ☐

Step 2: Think up a range of possible activities to overcome the specific reduced activity

> Muriel's problem is that she wants 'to start meeting up with people again'. She sits and thinks about things she could do to overcome her isolation. Muriel comes up with a range of possible things she could do to start meeting up with people again. Read Muriel's list below:
>
> ● *Have a party.*
>
> ● *Ask my sister Mary round again.*
>
> ● *Phone my friend Sarah.*

Step 3: Deciding which activity to do

One problem that often faces people when they have reduced what they do is that it can seem difficult to begin to start changing this. They look at things and think that they 'must' suddenly do everything, and this feels like too much so they don't do anything as a result. They need to decide on doing things at the right pace – in a step-by-step way.

The next step is to think about the advantages and disadvantages of each possible option.

Suggestion	Advantages	Disadvantages
1 Have a party and invite all the neighbours.	*I'd meet lots of people.*	*The idea is too scary. It would be too hard getting ready for it. I couldn't cope with it.*
2 Ask my sister Mary round again.	*I always used to enjoy her visits and I do miss her company.*	*That could be nice as long as she didn't stay too long. I do worry what she will think of me, though.*
3 Phone my friend Sarah.	*We used to get on well and enjoyed meeting each other.*	*I haven't spoken to her for ages and it would be difficult explaining why I have phoned now.*

Step 4: Choose one of the activities

Muriel decides to do option 2 – to ask her sister Mary round.

> This solution should be an option that fulfils the following two criteria:
>
> **a)** Is it helpful? Yes ✓ No ☐
>
> **b)** Is it achievable Yes ✓ No ☐

Step 5: Plan the steps needed to carry out the activity

Muriel's plan:

Muriel thinks about how she can apply the questions for effective change in deciding on her plan:

1   Will it be useful for understanding or changing how I am?
Yes. I've found out a lot about mind-reading. I know I do that a lot. Even though I worry what Mary will think of me, I think that it will be useful for me to face up to my worries and ask her to come over.

2   Is it a specific task so that I will know when I have done it?
I'm clear what I am going to do – I'll invite her round one afternoon in the next week.

3   Is it realistic: is it practical and achievable?

Is it realistic – yes, I could do that, she's been before. I feel a little bit nervous about it, but I think I am probably just mind-reading again.

4   Does it make clear *what* you are going to do and *when* you are going to do it?
I could phone Mary up now and arrange it. I will invite her for a specific afternoon, – this Tuesday at 2.00 p.m. for an hour.

5   Is it an activity that won't be easily blocked or prevented by practical problems?
Now then, what might block it? Maybe she won't be in when I phone. If so, I'll phone later. Perhaps she will be busy on Tuesdays, after all she has such a busy life. If so, I'll ask her to come another day. If she isn't able to come then, I'm not going to take it personally, instead I'm just going to ask her again for next week. The only other block that could prevent it is if I lose my nerve and think about cancelling her, but I think it will be all right. I'm usually feeling at my best in the afternoon. As long as I tell her that it's just for an hour to begin with I think that will be fine. I'm going to invite her right now.'

Muriel's plan successfully answers each of the questions for effective change:

The *questions for effective change*	**Muriel's plan:**	
Is the planned activity one that:		
1 Will be **useful** for understanding or changing how I am?	Yes ✓	No ☐
2 Is a **specific task** so that I will know when I have done it?	Yes ✓	No ☐
3 Is **realistic**: is it practical and achievable?	Yes ✓	No ☐
4 Makes clear **what** I am going to do and **when** I am going to do it?	Yes ✓	No ☐
5 Is an activity that won't be easily blocked or prevented by practical problems?	Yes ✓	No ☐

Muriel's goals are **clear, specific** and **realistic**. She knows **what** she is going to do and **when** she will do it. She has predicted potential blocks that might get in the way. This seems like a well-thought out and planned way to increase her activity levels.

Step 6: Carry out the planned activity

Muriel's Plan:

Muriel phones her sister who says she is delighted to hear from Muriel. She says she has been worried about how she is and wants to visit. They arrange to meet on the Tuesday afternoon.

Step 7: Review the outcome

Checklist:

Muriel fights off her negative predictions that it will be really embarrassing meeting again, and that her sister will ask lots of prying questions or be really upset to see her like this. In fact, none of these fears come true. Her sister and Muriel get on very well. She feels supported by what Mary says, and they arrange to meet again for slightly longer next week. Overall, Muriel realises that she gained some pleasure from meeting Mary, and a definite sense of achievement.

	Muriel's review:	
Q. Was the selected approach successful?	Yes ✓	No ☐
Q. Did it help Muriel to start meeting up with people again (the target problem)?	Yes ✓	No ☐
Q. Were there any disadvantages to using this approach?	Yes ☐	No ✓

Muriel's activity:

In this case, Muriel's plan went smoothly. Even if there are any problems, she could have learned from them and used these to improve her next attempt to increase her activity.

The example used shows how the technique might be applied to Muriel's situation. However, it also can be applied to alter **any** problem of reduced activity. You now have the option of practising this approach.

Section 3 Creating your own plan to increase your activity levels

The following table summarises activities that are commonly altered when someone becomes depressed. A wide range of altered behaviours have been summarised here to help you to think about the changes that may occur. It is likely that you will have noticed changes in at least some of these activities. Sometimes people are not at first aware of how their depression has affected them.

Think about each of these activities. How has depression affected your behaviour?

Problems of reduced activity	Present in my case? (tick if present)
Stopping meeting friends.	
Reducing socialising or going out.	
Reducing my hobbies/interests.	
Reducing a specific activity that led to a sense of pleasure.	
Reducing a specific activity that led to a sense of achievement.	
My life is becoming emptier.	
Other (write in):	

It is not possible to deal with every reduced activity all at once. In fact, if you try to change everything at once you will be potentially setting yourself up to fail. **Please select only *one problem of reduced activity from above* that you wish to change at the present time.**

Once you have chosen one target, write it down here. My target is:

In order to create a clear plan of how to slowly re-introduce activities which previously gave you a sense of pleasure and achievement, the key is to apply the principles you learned by looking at Muriel's plan.

Step 1: Clearly define your reduced activity that needs to be changed. Be as precise as possible

My reduced activity:

Q. Is this a clear, focused activity?   Yes ☐   No ☐

Step 2: Think up a range of possible activities to overcome the specific reduced activity

Think about things you can do to overcome your chosen reduced activity.

Write them in the box below:

Step 3: Deciding which activity to do

The next step is to think about the advantages and disadvantages of each possible option.

Suggestion	Advantages	Disadvantages

Step 4: Choose one of the activities

Decide on an option based upon what you have thought about in step 3.

This solution should be an option that fulfils the following two criteria:

a) Is it helpful?   Yes ☐   No ☐

b) Is it achievable   Yes ☐   No ☐

Step 5: Plan the steps needed to carry out the activity

My plan to increase my activity levels

✎ Write your plan down here.

Your task is to carry this out during the next week.

Check your plan against each of the questions for effective change.

The questions for effective change

Is my planned activity one that: **My plan:**

1   will be **useful** for understanding or changing how I am?   Yes ☐   No ☐

2   is a **specific task** so that I will know when I have done it?   Yes ☐   No ☐

3   is **realistic**: is it practical and achievable?   Yes ☐   No ☐

4   makes clear **what** I am going to do and **when** I am going to do it?   Yes ☐   No ☐

5   is an activity that won't be easily blocked or prevented by practical problems?   Yes ☐   No ☐

You should be able to answer 'yes' to each of the questions. If you have noticed that your current plan has failed on one of the questions, try to think why this is. What changes can you make to alter or improve it? Try to change or alter the activity so that any poorly planned aspects are improved.

Many people find this approach takes quite a lot of practice. It may also be tempting to be too ambitious. Before moving on, ask yourself again, whether this is a target activity that you can cope with at present. If not, swap it for a more realistic and smaller target. Remember, large changes can be achieved by moving one step at a time. Do not push yourself too hard by being overly ambitious.

If you can answer 'yes' to each of these five questions, it means that your activity is well planned out. Try to write down **exactly** what you will do and plan to put it into practice this week.

Step 6: Carry out the planned activity

My Plan:

Carry out your plan, and pay attention to your thoughts about what will happen before, during and after you have completed the activity.

Step 7: Review the outcome

My Review:

✎ Write what happened here:

My review:

Q. Was the selected approach successful?	Yes ☐	No ☐
Q. Did it help me to tackle the target problem?	Yes ☐	No ☐
Q. Were there any disadvantages to using this approach?	Yes ☐	No ☐

When you have completed your activity:

Look back and think about your planned activity.

Think in detail about how your planned activity went:

Q. How much of a sense of achievement did you feel *while doing* the task?

Very little ——————————————— Very much

0   10

If you noticed that the activity gave you a *high* sense of achievement at the time:

This is important because it shows that by altering your activity, you can also alter your sense of achievement in things. This can provide a powerful tool for overcoming depression. Your experience also shows that you have picked an effective activity to change because it led to this feeling.

If you noticed that the activity gave you *only a slight* sense of achievement at the time:

Try to think about the factors that robbed you of a higher sense of achievement at the time. Were you aware of any negative or undermining thoughts such as '*I should have done it anyway*' or '*It's a waste of time*'? You can learn how to identify and challenge unhelpful thoughts like these in workbooks 4 and 5. In the mean time, if thoughts such as these are present, please try to **stop, think and reflect** on them rather than immediately accepting them as being true.

Q. How much of a sense of pleasure did you experience *while doing* the task?

Very little ——————————————— Very much

0   10

If you noticed that the activity gave you a *high* sense of pleasure at the time:

This shows that by altering your activity you can improve how you feel. Trying to increase your activity levels in this area in a step-by-step way may be helpful in boosting your mood.

If you noticed that the activity gave you *only a slight* sense of pleasure at the time:

Try to think about the factors that prevented you from experiencing pleasure. Were you aware of any negative thoughts that undermined how you felt? Were you distracted by other concerns and therefore didn't allow yourself to stop, think and reflect on what you were doing? Sometimes, extreme and unhelpful statements or rules (such as *should, must, got to* and *ought* statements) may come into mind and undermine the person's pleasure in things. Did this happen to you?

Hint

Thinking back on the areas in the week that have been pleasurable can act to boost how you feel. Sometimes people keep a diary and record positive events such as conversations, activities etc. that have provided them with a sense of pleasure or achievement. Use this approach to try to develop a more helpful focus to your thinking. They then build in a time each day to reflect on these events and remember them. In other words they choose to focus and remember positive things.

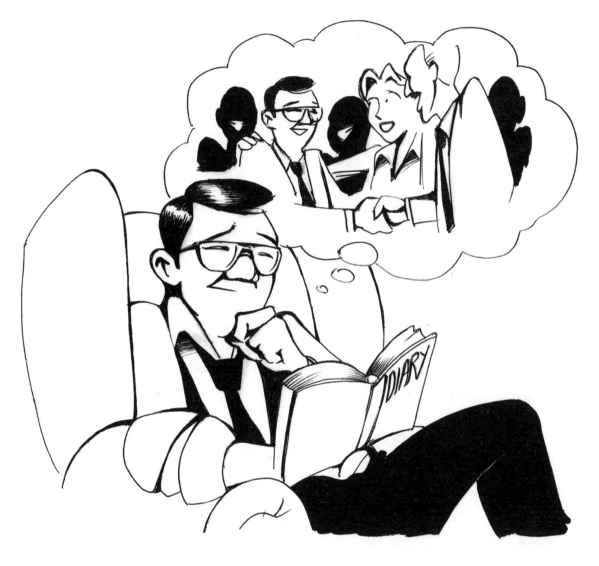

This idea of choosing to build in a **helpful focus** to at least part of your day can help boost mood. Try this approach to see if it is helpful for you. Decide to keep thinking from time to time about your achievements and take pleasure in what you have done.

Think again about how your target activity went:

Q. How easy was it for you to do the task?

Very difficult ——————————————————— Very easy

0   10

If it was fairly easy for you to do the task:

This shows that you chose to do an activity that you could successfully complete. Choosing realistic targets for change is important. Choosing activities that are focused and clear, and which you can succeed in is the key to effective change. Sometimes an activity can seem too easy. If this is the case, you have the option of choosing something that is a little harder next time. By making slow, sure steps you will be able to build your confidence and increase the things you do which give you a sense of pleasure and achievement.

If it was quite hard for you to do the task:

Choosing realistic targets for change is important. Sometimes it is tempting to choose an activity that is too ambitious. Instead, choose activities that are focused and clear, and which you can succeed in. By making slow, sure steps you will be able to build your confidence and increase the things you do which give you a sense of pleasure and achievement. Applying the *questions for effective change* can help you create a realistic action plan.

Q. Did any problems or difficulties occur in what you did?   Yes ☐   No ☐

If you had some difficulties in carrying out your planned activity:

This provides you with the opportunity to learn useful information for next time you plan an activity. Try to think about what happened. Could you have predicted the problem? What could you have done to prevent it? How could you put what you have learned into practice next time? Sometimes problems are unpredictable. If so, don't let yourself be put off trying this approach. Try it again. Use the problem as an opportunity to learn.

If you didn't have any difficulties in carrying out your planned activity:

It is good that there were no difficulties in carrying out your activity. It is likely that you had planned it well. Before planning any activity, it is important to consider whether it is realistic, and also to try to predict any possible blocks or difficulties. At some time when you do an activity, something may occur that will prevent you completing it. If that is the case, this provides you with the opportunity to learn useful information for next time. Try to think about what happened. Could you have predicted the problem? What could you have done to prevent it? How could you put what you have learned into practice next time? Use the problem as an opportunity to learn.

Section *4*   **Creating a further action plan**

Now that you have considered how your planned activity went, the next step is to plan another activity to put into practice over the next week or so. Use what you have just learned about how your activity went to build on what you did.

You have the choice to:

● repeat what you did;
● take what you did and move it on one stage further;
● or select a new area of activity.

There are advantages and disadvantages of each of these choices. Think about what the advantages and disadvantages may be for you.

Choosing a new target activity

Choices for the target activity	Advantages	Disadvantages
Repeat what you did.	Build confidence. Practise activity again. Overcome problems that occurred the first time.	If you found the task easy the first time, it is best to try to choose a more difficult activity.
Take what you did and move it on one stage further.	Step-by-step approach builds confidence in the chosen activity.	Your target activity must be realistic. Being too ambitious may lead you to give up or decide the activity isn't possible.
Or select a new area of activity.	Allows you to focus on another important activity.	The danger is moving from topic to topic and not making changes in any one activity area.

You must decide for yourself which decision is the best for you. It is not possible to deal with every problem activity all at once. In fact, if you try to change everything at once you will be potentially setting yourself up to fail.

Please select *one problem of reduced activity* that you wish to change at the present time.

Problems of reduced activity	Tick one activity only
Stopping meeting friends.	
Reducing socialising or going out.	
Reducing my hobbies/interests.	
Reducing a specific activity that led to a sense of pleasure.	
Reducing a specific activity that led to a sense of achievement.	
Other (write in):	

Once you have chosen one target reduced activity that you wish to change, write it down here. My target activity is:

In order to create a clear plan of how to slowly re-introduce activities that previously gave you a sense of pleasure and achievement, the key is to again create your own clear **action plan**. This will help you to practise and re-inforce your skills in creating this plan.

Do:

- plan to alter **only** one or two key activities over the next week.

- produce an **action plan** to slowly alter what you do in an effective and planned way.

- ask yourself the *questions for effective change* to check that your activity is well planned.

- write down your action plan in detail so that you will be able to put it into practice this week.

Don't:

- choose something that is too ambitious a target to start with.

- try to start to alter too many activities all at once.

- be very negative and think, *'nothing can be done'*, *'what's the point?'*, *'it's a waste of time'*. Try to experiment to find out if this negative thinking is wholly accurate or helpful.

✎ Write your action plan here:

Use what you have learned earlier to write your action plan. Plan what you will do and when you will do it. Learn from what happens so that you can keep putting what you have learned into practice. By doing this, you will be able to increase your activity levels in a planned, step-by-step way. By doing this, you will be slowly able to re-build your confidence, and increase your feelings of pleasure and achievement.

Section 5   **Workbook summary**

In this workbook you have:
- revised the vicious circle of reduced activity;
- seen an example of Muriel planning a way of increasing her activity levels;
- practised this approach yourself and reviewed how your planned activity went;
- planned a further activity to put into practice.

Putting what you have learned into practice

Please can you carry out a series of **action plans** over the next few weeks to overcome reduced activity in order to give you a sense of pleasure or achievement. Do not try to do everything all at once, but plan out what to do at a pace that is right for you. Discuss this with your health care practitioner if you are stuck or unsure what to do.

My notes

....

....

....

....

....

....

....

....

....

....

....

....

....

....

....

....

....

....

....

....

....

....

....

....

My notes

....

Workbook 7

Changing altered behaviours: unhelpful behaviours

Dr Chris Williams

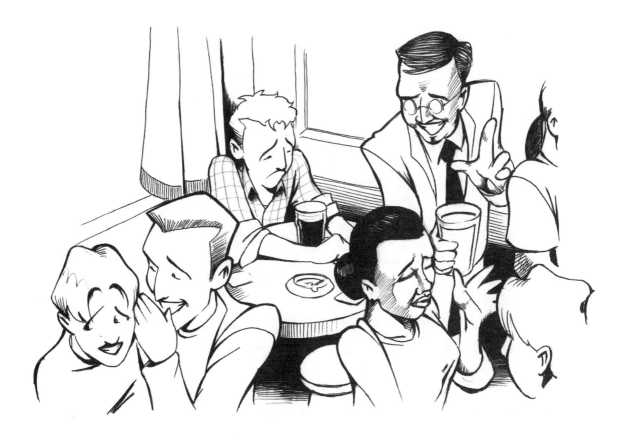

Overcoming Depression
A Five Areas Approach

Section 1 **Introduction**

In this workbook you will:

- revise the vicious circle of unhelpful behaviours;
- learn some brief hints and tips of ways to reduce unhelpful behaviours;
- practise a structured approach to plan a reduction in an unhelpful behaviour;
- answer a series of questions to see whether your level of drinking may be mentally and physically worsening how you feel.

In workbook 1 (*Understanding depression*), you looked at how depression may result in a *vicious circle of unhelpful behaviours*: starting (or increasing) behaviours that might act to worsen your depression and keep you depressed. This might include starting drinking, becoming very dependent on others, trying to spend your way out of depression, etc. This is the target for change within the current workbook.

When somebody becomes depressed, it is normal for him or her to alter their behaviour to try and get better.

Helpful activities may include:

- talking to friends for support;

- reading or using self-help materials to find out more about the causes and treatment of depression;

- going to see their doctor or health care practitioner to discuss what treatments may be helpful;

- maintaining activities that give pleasure such as meeting friends, etc.

Sometimes however, the person may try to block how they feel by using unhelpful behaviours e.g.:

- withdrawing into themselves and cutting themselves off from all their friends;

- using alcohol to block how they feel;

- neglecting themselves (e.g. by not eating as much);

- harming themselves as a way of blocking how they feel (e.g. self-cutting).

A **vicious circle of unhelpful behaviours can result.**

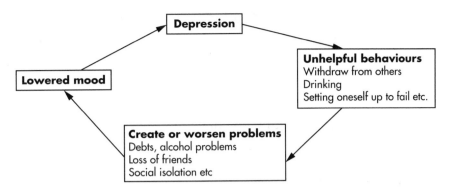

Figure 7.1 The vicious circle of unhelpful behaviour

My unhelpful behaviours

Please look at the following questions and **tick yes** if you have found yourself doing these things in the last week.

Q. Am I misusing alcohol to block how I feel?	Yes ☐	No ☐
Q. Am I misusing other substances such as illegal drugs?	Yes ☐	No ☐
Q. Am I becoming excessively clingy and dependent?	Yes ☐	No ☐
Q. Am I becoming very suspicious and demanding?	Yes ☐	No ☐
Q. Am I setting myself up to fail?	Yes ☐	No ☐
Q. Am I setting myself up to be let down or rejected?	Yes ☐	No ☐
Q. Am I trying to spend my way out of depression?	Yes ☐	No ☐

✎ Other (write in)

Q. Overall, do unhelpful behaviours have an unhelpful effect on me? Yes ☐   No ☐

Section 2 Hints and tips for dealing with unhelpful behaviours

The following questions ask about some common unhelpful behaviours and provide some hints and tips to help change these:

Q. Are you misusing tablets such as illegal drugs? Yes ☐ No ☐

Misusing tablets such as illegal drugs can worsen symptoms of depression and may prevent you getting better. This is especially true of cocaine, amphetamines and heroin.

Important task

If you are using illegal substances on a regular basis, this may act to prevent you getting better. If you are using these drugs, we strongly suggest that you discuss this with your health care practitioner, who will be able to advise you how to help cut down and stop your substance misuse.

Q. Are you becoming very suspicious and demanding? Yes ☐ No ☐

Try to be at least a little less demanding of others. If you have been saying unhelpful comments to others, try to reduce them. It will not help you or others to be very demanding of them. By holding back, you will begin to build up your trust in others, and also they will find it easier to offer you support. The best way of overcoming the concerns or worries that might be driving your suspicion is to undermine them by choosing not to act on them. At first this may be quite difficult.

Q. Are you setting yourself up to fail? Yes ☐ No ☐

This is an important pattern of behaviour to notice because it is likely that it will continue to keep you feeling low in mood and may reinforce beliefs of failure. Try to look for this pattern of behaviour, and if it is present ask yourself – *'Do I really benefit by doing this?'* Try not to set yourself up to fail because it is likely that these actions will reinforce underlying beliefs of failure or incompetency and thus act to keep your depression going.

Q. Are you setting yourself up to be let down or rejected? Yes ☐ No ☐

This behaviour is likely to keep you feeling low in mood. It may reinforce thoughts of rejection. Try to look for this pattern of behaviour, and ask yourself – *'Is this really helpful?'* These actions will reinforce underlying beliefs of unlovability or worthlessness and thus act to keep your depression going. Try to act against this pattern by stopping doing actions that may lead you to be let down or rejected in this way.

Q. Are you trying to spend your way out of depression? Yes ☐ No ☐

This can be very expensive and doesn't work. It can also create a new range of practical problems as a result of debt. Practical changes such as avoiding carrying too much money with you when you shop and leaving your credit cards at home may help in the short term. You could also plan what you are going to buy in advance so there are no impulse buys. In the longer term though, you need to find more effective ways of overcoming your depression than spending your way out of it.

Alcohol – a potentially unhelpful behaviour

Alcohol can sometimes be misused. In small doses, drink can make the person feel more relaxed and block out worries. If taken at larger doses for a number of weeks or months it can cause a number of important problems.

The recommended highest levels of alcohol to be taken *each week* are:

- 22 units for women, and

- 28 units for men.

Useful information: 1 unit is half a pint of bitter or lager, or 1 glass of wine, or one measure of spirits. These values vary, so strong lagers or beers, or fortified wines, etc. will contain far more than one unit of alcohol.

Q. How many units of alcohol do you drink a week: ✎ . . . . units

---

Choice point

If you drink more than the recommended levels, please answer the following questions. Otherwise, move to section 4.

Section 3   **The impact of alcohol on you**

Alcohol at high levels can cause a range of problems. Think about the following areas and then answer the questions.

Thinking changes as a result of alcohol:

- High levels of alcohol can worsen depression and prevent recovery.

- It can worsen worry and panic attacks.

- It can lead to acute bouts of confusion or violence in drunkenness.

- It can cause the person to become increasingly suspicious and paranoid.

- It can lead to psychological addiction with craving if abruptly stopped.

Q Do you have any of these mental symptoms?   Yes ☐   No ☐

Physical changes as a result of alcohol:

- Alcohol can lead to physical addiction with withdrawal symptoms such as sweatiness and sickness if abruptly stopped. This is called **alcohol dependency**.

- It can cause damage to parts of the body (for example causing stomach ulcers, cirrhosis of the liver, epileptic fits or damage to important body organs such as the pancreas).

Q. Do you have any of these physical symptoms?   Yes ☐   No ☐

Social changes as a result of alcohol:

- It can cause problems at home such as arguments with family and friends.

- It can lead to debts.

- It can lead to mistakes at work, arriving late etc. that can lead to difficulties at work.

- Accidents, violence and car crashes are all common social consequences of alcohol dependency.

Q. Do you have any of these social symptoms?   Yes ☐   No ☐

Alcohol dependency means that the body and mind become so used to the presence of alcohol, that if alcohol is suddenly completely stopped or is reduced too quickly, a range of withdrawal symptoms can occur. These might include sleeplessness, irritability, sweatiness, sickness, headaches and at its extreme, confusion, hallucinations and very serious physical illness which requires urgent medical assessment and treatment.

Q. Overall, do you believe that you are experiencing drink problems?   Yes ☐   No ☐

Thank you for answering these questions. **If you are drinking to excess,** unless you can reduce the amount you drink, you are likely to cause yourself increasing problems in each of these areas. You need to tackle your drinking problem **now**. You may be tempted to downplay or ignore your drinking and believe it is not a problem. This is often part of the problem of excessive drinking. Please discuss this with your health care practitioner.

Important task

If you are regularly drinking more than **22 units of alcohol a week (women)** or **28 units (men),** and less than 49 units/week, this is higher than the recommended healthy alcohol intake. If this is the case, then you need to try to cut down the amount you drink. Try to reduce your overall drinking each week. Build in at least two days without any drink to allow your body to recover. Discuss how best to do this with your health care practitioner.

Important task

If your drinking is **above 50 units/week,** this is **well above** the healthy drink range. If you stop drinking completely now, it is possible that you will notice some symptoms of withdrawal. Please try to cut down the amount you drink in a slow step-by-step manner. If you do not do this, it is unlikely that you will quickly get over your feelings of depression. Discuss how best to do this with your health care practitioner.

Section *4* Overcoming unhelpful behaviours

By working through the seven steps outlined below you can learn an approach that will help you to plan clear ways of overcoming your unhelpful behaviours.

Example: Problems of excessive drink

Paul is a 35 year old man who is depressed. He has continued to work in his office job, but has felt lower and lower in confidence. He has begun to drink every day *'to steady my nerves'*. He is now drinking around 20 pints (40 units) of beer a week, which is well above the recommended healthy alcohol range for a man. He is becoming worried that he will become addicted to the drink, and decides he wants to *'do something about it'*.

Compare his plan *'to do something about it'* against **the** *questions for effective change*:

The questions for effective change	Paul's plan	
1 Will it be useful for understanding or changing how he is?	Yes ☐	No ✓
2 Is it a **specific task** so that he will know when he has done it?	Yes ☐	No ✓
3 Is it **realistic**: is it practical and achievable for him?	Yes ☐	No ✓
4 Does it make clear **what** he is going to do and **when** he is going to do it?	Yes ☐	No ✓
5 Is it an activity that won't be easily blocked or prevented by practical problems?	Yes ☐	No ✓

His goal is **not specific** enough. It does not tell Paul **what** to do nor defines the steps needed to reach the goal. Because of this, the plan fails the *questions for effective change* test. Poorly defined plans do not address the questions **'What am I going to do?'** and **'When am I going to do it?'** and Paul's goals therefore need to change in order to help him have a clearer plan of what to do.

Paul's first task is to decide on a specific plan to reduce his unhelpful drinking. He does this by using a seven step approach to reducing his unhelpful behaviour.

Step 1: Clearly define the unhelpful behaviour that needs to be reduced. Be as precise as possible

Paul's unhelpful behaviour:
I am drinking 20 pints a week. I want to cut this down so that I am not drinking as much.
Q. Is this a clear, focused unhelpful behaviour?   Yes ✓   No ☐

Step 2: Paul thinks up a range of ways to slowly reduce his specific unhelpful behaviour

Think about things you can do to overcome your chosen problem. Write them in the box below:

- *I could give up drinking immediately.*

- *I could slowly reduce what I drink.*

- *I could go away on holiday somewhere where I can't buy drink.*

- *I could join Alcoholics Anonymous.*

Step 3: Deciding how to reduce his unhelpful behaviour

The next step is to think about the advantages and disadvantages of each possible option.

Suggestion	Advantages	Disadvantages
1 I could give up drinking immediately.	*I wouldn't be drinking.*	*I've been told by my doctor that I might have some symptoms of alcohol withdrawal.*
2 I could slowly reduce what I drink.	*It would mean that I could plan a slow reduction – this might work.*	*I'd need to have a good plan. I've tried this before and quickly given up.*
3 I could go away on holiday somewhere where I can't buy drink.	*It would be nice to get away from it all.*	*I can't afford to go away. I bet I'd drink there anyway.*
4 I could join Alcoholics Anonymous.	*Others might encourage me to give up. It would be good to know I'm not on my own.*	*I don't want to do this. I want to try on my own at the moment.*

Step 4: Choose one of the plans

Decide on an option based upon what you have thought about in step 3.

Paul decides on option 2, and to do this with help and advice from his health care practitioner. This solution should be an option that fulfils the two criteria of being helpful and achievable:

a) Is it helpful? Yes ✓ No ☐

b) Is it achievable? Yes ✓ No ☐

Step 5: Plan the steps needed to carry out the reduction in the unhelpful behaviour

---

My plan to reduce my unhelpful behaviour

Paul's Target: 'I could slowly reduce what I drink.'

Paul thinks about how he can apply the questions for effective change in deciding on his plan:

1 Will it be useful for understanding or changing how I am?

Yes. I could learn that I can cut it down, if I use the right plan.

2 Is it a specific task so that I will know when I have done it?

I'm clear what I am going to do – I want to have cut down to 10 pints a week. That will be my target.

3 Is it realistic: is it practical and achievable?

Yes, I could cut to 10 pints. I don't want to stop completely, but that seems realistic.

4 Does it make clear *what* you are going to do and *when* you are going to do it?

I need to make sure I don't try and rush things. My doctor told me that I might have withdrawal problems if I stop drinking too quickly. If I cut back by 2 pints every other day, I can be down to 10 pints in 5 days. That seems a bit fast – I might not be able to manage that. It would be better to cut by one pint every 2 days – so I could do it in 20 days. That's a bit longer than I originally thought, but I think that will be a better plan.

5 Is it an activity that won't be easily blocked or prevented by practical problems?

What could prevent this? I'm due to go to Bob's party next Saturday. There's bound to be drinking there – I'd need to set myself a limit of maybe 2 pints on that day. I could tell them I'm driving. I also need to stop buying in six packs for the time being – they are too tempting when I am feeling low. The most I'll buy now is two cans. That should help because I know that when I've had one can, I often have a few more.

Check the plan against each of the questions for effective change.

The *questions for effective change*		Paul's plan:	
Is the planned changed activity one that:			
1 Will be **useful** for understanding or changing how I am?		Yes ✓	No ☐
2 Is a **specific task** so that I will know when I have done it?		Yes ✓	No ☐
3 Is **realistic**: is it practical and achievable?		Yes ✓	No ☐
4 Makes clear **what** I am going to do and **when** I am going to do it?		Yes ✓	No ☐
5 Is an activity that won't be easily blocked or prevented by practical problems?		Yes ✓	No ☐

Step 6: Carry out the plan to reduce the unhelpful behaviour

Paul puts his plan into practice over the next 20 days.

Step 7: Review the outcome

Paul's review:

Write what happened here:

Paul manages to put his plan into action for the first few days and he feels quite good about himself and how things are going. Things don't go according to plan, though, when Paul goes to Bob's party. He has two cans to drink, and then thinks 'what the heck, let your hair down'. He ends up drinking ten pints in a binge and has to get a taxi home. The next day he wakes up feeling worse and thinks about giving up the planned reduction in drinking completely. After a few hours, he begins to think about what he has learned before from his doctor about having to stick to a clear plan if he is going to succeed. He also remembers his doctor telling him that it is likely there will be occasional hiccups, but that can work out for the good – he can learn from what happens and plan to avoid making the same mistake again. Just because a set-back occurs does not mean that everything is over. Paul therefore tries again and restarts his plan. He finds that he is able to reach his target of drinking 10 pints a week over the next few weeks.

Paul's review:

Q. Was the selected approach successful?	Yes ✓	No ☐
Q. Did it help me to tackle the target problem?	Yes ✓	No ☐
Q. Were there any disadvantages to using this approach?	Yes ☐	No ✓

The example used shows how the technique might be applied to Paul's situation. However, it also can be applied to alter **any** unhelpful activity. You now have the option of practising this approach.

Section 5 Overcoming your unhelpful behaviour

7.12

Apply what you have learned from Paul's example, and answer the questions below.

Step 1: Clearly define the unhelpful behaviour that needs to be reduced. Be as precise as possible

My unhelpful behaviour:

Q. Is this a clear, focused problem behaviour?   Yes ☐   No ☐

Step 2: Think up a range of ways to slowly reduce the specific unhelpful behaviour

Think about things you can do to overcome your unhelpful behaviour. ✎Write them in the box below:

Step 3: Deciding how to reduce the unhelpful behaviour

The next step is to think about the advantages and disadvantages of each possible option.

Suggestion	Advantages	Disadvantages

Step 4: Choose one of the plans

Decide on an option based upon what you have found in step 3.

This solution should be an option that fulfils the following two criteria:

a) Is it helpful? Yes ☐ No ☐

b) Is it achievable? Yes ☐ No ☐

My option:

Step 5: Plan the steps needed to carry out the reduction in the unhelpful behaviour

My plan to reduce my unhelpful behaviour

✎ Write your plan down here.

Your task is to carry this out during the next week.

Check your plan against each of the questions for effective change.

The *questions for effective change*	My plan:	
Is my plan to reduce my unhelpful behaviour one that:		
1 Will be **useful** for understanding or changing how I am?	Yes ☐	No ☐
2 Is a **specific task** so that I will know when I have done it?	Yes ☐	No ☐
3 Is **realistic**: is it practical and achievable?	Yes ☐	No ☐
4 Makes clear **what** I am going to do and **when** I am going to do it?	Yes ☐	No ☐
5 Is an activity that won't be easily blocked or prevented by practical problems?	Yes ☐	No ☐

Step 6: Carry out the plan to reduce the unhelpful behaviour

Step 7: Review the outcome

My Review:

✎ Write what happened here:

| |
| |

	My review:	
Q. Was the selected approach successful?	Yes ☐	No ☐
Q. Did it help me to reduce the unhelpful behaviour?	Yes ☐	No ☐
Q. Were there any disadvantages to using this approach?	Yes ☐	No ☐

Think again about how your plan to reduce the unhelpful behaviour went:

Q. How easy was it for you to reduce the unhelpful behaviour?

Very difficult ——————————————————— Very easy

0   10

If it was fairly easy:

This shows that you chose something that you could successfully complete. Choosing realistic targets for change is important. Sometimes the plan can seem too easy. If this is the case, you have the option of choosing something that is a little harder next time.

If it was quite hard:

Choosing realistic targets for change is important. Sometimes it is tempting to choose a target that is too ambitious. Instead, choose activities that are focused and clear, and which you can succeed in. By making slow, sure steps you will be able to build your confidence. Applying the *questions for effective change* can help you create a realistic action plan.

Q. Did any problems or difficulties occur in what you did?   Yes ☐   No ☐

If you had some difficulties in carrying out your planned activity:

This provides you with the opportunity to learn useful information for next time. Try to think about what happened. Could you have predicted the problem? What could you have done to prevent it? How could you put what you have learned into practice next time? Sometimes problems are unpredictable. If so, don't let yourself be put off trying this approach. Try it again. Use the problem as an opportunity to learn.

If you didn't have any difficulties in carrying out your planned activity:

This is probably because you had planned it well. At some time, something that you haven't planned may stop your plan to reduce the unhelpful behaviour. If so, try to learn from it. Could you have predicted the problem? What could you have done to prevent it? How could you put what you have learned into practice next time? Use the problem as an opportunity to learn.

Creating a further action plan

You will need to slowly build on what you have done in a step-by-step way. You have the choice to:

- stick at the target you have achieved;
- focus on the same unhelpful behaviour but plan to reduce it further;
- or select a new unhelpful behaviour to reduce.

There are advantages and disadvantages of each of these choices. Think about what the advantages and disadvantages may be for you.

Choosing a new unhelpful behaviour to reduce

Choices for the target activity	Advantages	Disadvantages
Stick at the level you have achieved	You may be happy with this. The key is whether the behaviour is still at a level that is harming you or others.	You have to plan so that the level of behaviour doesn't drift up again.
Focus on the same unhelpful behaviour but plan to reduce it further	Step-by-step approach will allow you to make progress over time.	Your target must be realistic. Being too ambitious may lead you to give up.
Or select a new activity area	Allows you to focus on another area you think is important.	The danger is moving from topic to topic and not maintaining changes in any one area.

You must decide for yourself which decision is the best for you. It is not possible to deal with every unhelpful behaviour at once. In fact, if you try to change everything at once you will be potentially setting yourself up to fail.

Section 6 **Workbook summary**

In this workbook, you have:

● revised the vicious circle of unhelpful behaviours;

● learned some brief hints and tips of ways to reduce unhelpful behaviours;

● practiced a structured approach to plan a reduction in an unhelpful behaviour;

● answered a series of questions to see whether your level of drinking may be mentally and physically worsening how you feel (optional).

Putting what you have learned into practice

Please can you carry out the **action plan** that you created earlier to reduce one unhelpful behaviour over the next week. Do not try to do everything all at once, but plan out what to do at a pace that is right for you. Discuss this with your health care practitioner if you are stuck or unsure what to do.

Important task

If you are regularly using illegal substances or drinking excessive alcohol, please can you discuss this with your health care practitioner. If you are doing this on a regular basis, this may act to prevent you getting better.

My notes

....

....

....

....

....

....

....

....

....

....

....

....

....

....

....

....

....

....

....

....

....

....

My notes

....

Workbook 8
Overcoming sleep and other problems

Dr Chris Williams

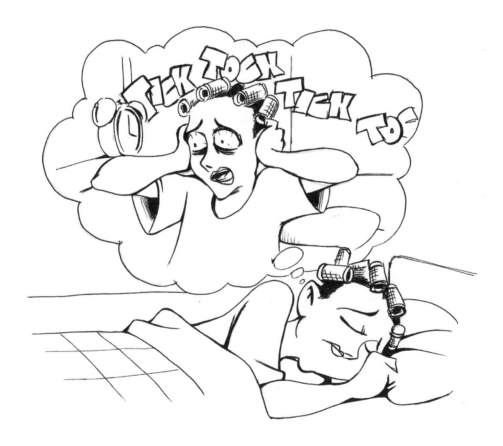

Overcoming Depression
A Five Areas Approach

Section *1* **Introduction**

In this workbook you will learn:
- what are sleep and insomnia;
- common causes of sleep problems and actions you can take to help overcome problems of poor sleep;
- hints and tips for overcoming common physical problems that occur as part of depression.

Understanding sleep problems

Sleeping problems are common and affect large numbers of people. At times, sleep can be disrupted for a variety of different reasons.

What is sleep?

In spite of the fact that we spend around a third of our lives asleep, sleep is something that we often take for granted until we are unable to do it. The amount of sleep each individual needs varies throughout their life. Babies and young children need a lot more sleep than older adults. Many people find that by the time they reach their 60s or 70s, the amount of sleep they need has dropped by up to several hours a day. The average time we sleep is often said to be about eight hours but this is only true for some people. There is a wide normal healthy sleep range. Some people sleep only four to six hours a day whereas others can sleep for as many as 10 or 12 hours a day. Both extremes are quite normal.

What is insomnia?

Insomnia, or inability to sleep, is something that many people notice from time to time. Insomnia may start after an isolated incident or an upsetting life event, or it can be related to a feature of a person's lifestyle. Think about the following factors that can worsen sleep and see whether they are present in your own life.

Factors affecting sleep

Preparing for sleep

The time leading up to sleep can be very important. Try to build in a '**wind-down**' time when you are less active. Physical over-activity (e.g. exercising), or eating too much just before bed may keep you awake. Sometimes people read in bed, or watch television while lying in bed. This sometimes can help them wind down, but for many people it can make them become more alert – therefore adding to sleep problems.

Q. Am I engaging in activities, which wake me up when I should be winding down? Yes ☐   No ☐

If yes: Try to avoid watching television or working in bed. Try to keep your bed as a place for sleep or sex. Try to avoid lying on your bed reading, working or worrying. This will only cause your brain to become overactive and prevent you sleeping. You need to decide for yourself whether listening to a radio or music is conducive to sleep or not in your particular case.

If you are taking part in a keep fit programme, this is a good thing, however it is best to take exercise no later than the early evening. Try to avoid doing exercise in the half-hour before going to sleep as it may backfire and wake you up.

Physical problems

Sometimes symptoms such as pain, itching or other physical symptoms can cause sleeplessness. Tackling these physical symptoms may be an effective treatment of your insomnia.

Q. Are physical symptoms keeping me awake? Yes ☐   No ☐

If yes: If physical symptoms such as itching or pain are keeping you awake, please discuss this with your doctor or health care practitioner. Sometimes symptoms of depression can worsen symptoms such as pain, in which case treating the depression will help to reduce the pain.

Physical environment

Think about the conditions where you sleep. Is your bed comfortable? If possible you should try to change your mattress at least every eight to ten years. What about the temperature of the room where you sleep? If the room is either very cold or very hot this might make sleeping difficult.

Is the room very noisy? Sometimes it is easier to get off to sleep if the room or house where you live is quiet. Although noise can keep people awake, it is often short-term noises that occur intermittently that are more likely to cause awakening than more long-term droning noises. Is there too much light to sleep? If bright lights such as streetlights come through your curtains, this can sometimes prevent sleep.

Q. Do I try and sleep in a poor sleep environment Yes ☐   No ☐

If yes: The following are specific things that you can do to overcome a poor sleep environment:

- **Poor mattress**: If your mattress is old, change it if you can. If not, try turning it over, or rotate it. Sometimes adding additional supports such as a board underneath it can help.

- **Too hot/cold**: If it is too hot, alter the ventilation. Open a window or use a fan. If it is too cold, think about insulation (many grants are available), secondary or double-glazing etc., or add an extra blanket.

- **Problems with noise**: Reduce external noise. Think about tackling the causes of noise directly. Can you speak to noisy neighbours and ask them to turn down their music? Have you thought about fitting double-glazing or internal plastic sheeting over windows to reduce noise? Sometimes purchasing a white noise generator, which produces a monotonous low-level noise, can mask intrusive external sounds.

- **Problems with excessive light**: Consider changing your curtains; adding a thicker lining (or blackout lining) can help. If cost is a problem, a black plastic bin bag can also be an effective blackout blind if stapled or stuck to the curtain rail.

Psychological problems

A range of different psychological problems such as anxiety, depression, and worry or stress at work or in relationships can upset sleep. For example, a person who suffers from depression may find that it takes them up to several hours to get off to sleep. They may then experience a disrupted sleep pattern with multiple awakenings, and then finally wake up several hours earlier than normal feeling unrested or on edge. Treatment of the depression will lead to an improvement in the quality of sleep.

Similarly, problems of anxiety and agitation can worsen sleep. In sleep, there is a reduction in arousal and tension levels leading the body and brain to begin to relax and drop off to sleep. In contrast, in worry, the brain becomes overly alert. The person is preoccupied by worrying thoughts and ends up mulling over things again and again in their mind. This is the exact opposite of what is needed to get off to sleep and can **cause** problems of insomnia.

Q. Do I notice anxiety and worry when I try to sleep?   Yes ☐   No ☐

Worry is often associated with a triggering of the body's **fight or flight adrenaline response**. This can cause the person to feel fidgety or restless and they may notice symptoms such as an increased heart rate, breathing rate, a churning stomach or tension throughout the body.

Q. Do I notice symptoms of depression when I try to sleep?   Yes ☐   No ☐

Depression is a common cause of sleeplessness. Treatment of depression can often be helpful in aiding sleep when this is the result of depression.

What about caffeine?

Caffeine is a chemical that is found in coffee, tea, cola drinks, hot chocolate and some herbal drinks. Caffeine causes increased alertness, an increased heart rate and if taken at high levels for several weeks can begin to cause physical and psychological dependence and symptoms of addiction. It may surprise you to know that drinking five strong cups of coffee a day on a regular basis has been shown to be physically addictive and also to reduce sleep quality. There is a danger that a vicious cycle can occur where tiredness causes the person to drink more coffee to keep alert, and then the coffee itself prevents the person obtaining the sleep that would have reduced the original tiredness.

Q. Am I drinking too much caffeine?   Yes ☐   No ☐

Try to avoid chemical stimulants. If you are regularly drinking more than five cups of strong coffee a day, you should try to either reduce your total caffeine intake in a step-by-step manner (e.g. by reducing by one cup of coffee a day), or switch to decaffeinated coffees or teas. Other caffeine-containing drinks should also be reduced if you are drinking them to excess. This will help your sleep, and also may reduce your general tension levels.

Avoid having a night-time cup of coffee or a last cigarette before sleep. Both caffeine and nicotine will keep you awake. Some people have found that taking a warm milky drink such as a bran-based drink can help you get off to sleep.

What about alcohol?

Sometimes people drink alcohol to reduce feelings of tension or depression or to help them get off to sleep. Studies have shown that if you drink more than the recommended levels of alcohol (22 units a week for women and 28 units for men, where one unit is approximately half a pint of beer, one short, or one glass of wine), symptoms such as anxiety, depression and sleeplessness can occur. In addition, if you drink too much of any liquid late at night you may find yourself having to make frequent visits to the toilet thus further keeping you awake.

Q. Am I drinking too much alcohol?　　　　　　　　Yes ☐　　No ☐

Getting up in the night to use the toilet can be avoided by reducing the amount of alcohol or other fluids you drink before going to bed. If you take a diuretic (a water tablet), you should try to take these earlier in the day to avoid having to get up during the night. Discuss this with your doctor.

　　If your drinking of alcohol is above the **healthy drink range**, please try to cut down the amount you drink in a slow step-by-step manner. If you do not do this, it is unlikely that you will quickly get over your feelings of depression or sleeplessness. Discuss how best to do this with your health care practitioner.

What about your sleep pattern?

Scientists have studied the brain to find out what happens during sleep. Like plants and animals we are affected by our surroundings and respond to rhythmic changes such as day and night. It is the cycle of day and night, light and dark that triggers our sleep pattern. Our **biological clock** is set by the natural daylight and night-time darkness that occurs each day. Sometimes when people don't sleep they disrupt their entire social calendar in an attempt to overcome this. Instead of going to sleep at a reasonable time, they may go to bed either **very much earlier** than normal or **very much later.** **Napping** is another habit that can end up backfiring by upsetting the natural sleep-wake cycle. This can cause great difficulties by altering the stability of the sleep pattern.

Q. Do I have a disrupted sleep pattern (time to bed/getting up)?　Yes ☐　　No ☐

If yes: Set yourself regular sleep times. Get up at a set time even if you have slept poorly. Try to teach your body what time to fall asleep and what time to get up. Try to go to sleep some time between 10 p.m. and midnight. Also make sure that you get up at a **sensible** time (preferably some time between 7 a.m. and 9 a.m.). Adjust these times appropriately to fit your own circumstances, however, it is advisable not to go to sleep either too early or to lie in bed too late in the morning. If you find you cannot get off to sleep, one helpful approach is to get up, do something else until you feel 'sleepy tired', and then return to bed.

Q. Do I nap during the day?　　　　　　　　　　Yes ☐　　No ☐

If yes: Teach your body clock a regular sleep/wake cycle. Avoid napping – taking naps in the day reduces the amount of sleep you need at night and can disrupt the need for night-time sleep. Daytime naps can cause sleep problems. It is important to try to avoid them.

Anxiety and insomnia are often linked together. Stress about life and about not sleeping contributes to insomnia. Extreme and catastrophic fears about not being able to sleep at all and therefore not being able to function with any efficiency can itself cause increased stress thus preventing the person getting off to sleep. The altered behaviour that is the result of this worry may actually end up worsening the problem. The key to the problem is **worry**. The impact of worry in causing and maintaining insomnia is summarised as the **vicious circle of insomnia**.

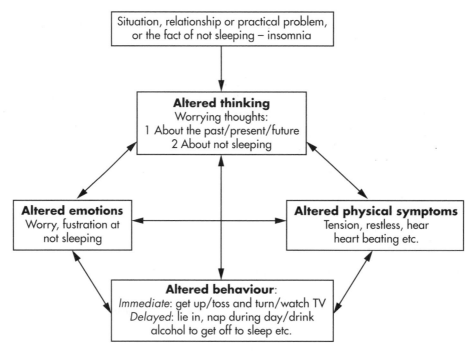

Figure 8.1 The vicious circle of insomnia.

The treatment of sleeplessness

Psychological treatment approaches to help people with sleeplessness depend on the **modification of worry**. Worry can be both a **cause and an effect** of poor sleep. Challenging extreme and catastrophic fears about the consequences of not sleeping is important. You can find out how to do this within workbooks 4 and 5. In addition, making changes to what you do when you don't sleep is important. One effective approach is to get up out of bed if you are not sleeping after 30 minutes, go downstairs and do something else until you are 'sleepy tired' again. Then return to bed.

Tackling worry about not sleeping

Worry about the consequences of not sleeping is very common. Common fears are that the person's performance at home or at work will plummet. Sometimes the person fears that they will become irritable and unable to cope. Sometimes they worry that either their brain or their body will be harmed by a lack of sleep.

This vicious circle of insomnia can be broken at a number of different places by:

- optimising conditions for sleep using the techniques described on the recent pages – this includes altering unhelpful behaviours that are maintaining the problem;
- reducing worry by learning a relaxation technique;
- challenging the extreme and unhelpful catastrophic thoughts about the consequences of a lack of sleep.

Important information about sleep

Sleep is a necessary part of life, however studies have shown that most people do not need very much sleep at all to be physically and mentally healthy. In sleep research laboratories, it has been found that many people who suffer from insomnia actually sleep far more than they think. Sometimes people who are actually sleeping and are in a light level of sleep can actually **be dreaming that they are awake**. This information may help allay fears that you are not sleeping at all. It is also important to know that sleep deprivation does **not** have catastrophic impacts on the brain or body. It is possible to function effectively with very little sleep each night.

Q. Do I have extreme or catastrophic fears about the consequences of not sleeping? Yes ☐   No ☐

Extreme and catastrophic fears can themselves **cause** increased wakefulness thus preventing you getting off to sleep. Being aware that these thoughts are extreme, inaccurate and unhelpful is important. Although you might feel tired and irritable, this does not necessarily affect your ability to perform tasks around the house or at work.

Key advice: Overcoming sleep difficulties

1   Try to get into a **routine**. Go to bed and get up at a regular time. Avoid drinking too much coffee, tea, hot chocolate and soft drinks, which contain caffeine – around five cups or glasses a day of caffeine-containing drinks should be the maximum. Switch to decaffeinated drinks or water for drinks beyond this.

2   **Nicotine** in cigarettes can also cause sleeplessness. Avoid smoking just before bed.

3   **Avoid napping** during the day. It upsets your body clock.

4   Watch your **alcohol** intake. Alcohol causes sleep to be shallow and unrefreshing and can cause you to waken to use the toilet.

5   Consider the **surroundings** to your sleep (noise, light levels, temperature, e.g. too hot or cold, and also the comfort of your bed).

6   If you don't get off to sleep, **get up, leave your bedroom** until you feel 'sleepy tired', then go to bed again.

Section 2 Hints and tips for overcoming common physical changes in depression

The following is a short practical summary of some immediate changes that you can bring about that may help the physical symptoms you are experiencing.

Physical symptoms of depression	Hints and tips
Difficulties getting off to sleep	1 Try to get into a **routine**. Go to bed and get up at a regular time. 2 **Avoid napping** during the day: it upsets your body clock. 3 Avoid drinking too much coffee, tea, hot chocolate and or soft drinks which contain caffeine – around five cups or glasses a day is the maximum. Switch to decaffeinated drinks if you drink more than this. 4 Watch your **alcohol** intake. Alcohol causes sleep to be shallow and unrefreshing.
Wakening earlier than usual	This is common in depression and improves as the depression gets better. 1 Try to rest in bed. 2 If you feel agitated get up. Consider medication to reduce agitation if this is a problem. Discuss this with your doctor. 3 Try to get up before 9.00 a.m. 4 If you lie in (or nap during the day), this is likely to upset your body clock and add to your problems.
A disrupted sleep pattern	1 Sleep problems are common in depression. They will not cause any immediate harm to your body or your mind. 2 If you find yourself waking up repeatedly during the night, get up, do something else (e.g. read, watch television but avoid scary films that may wake you up still further) until you feel 'sleepy tired', then go to bed again. **It is important not to sleep or nap during the next day** even if you feel tired.
A decreased appetite	1 Eating a balanced range of foods is important to keep both your physical and mental strength up. 2 Try to eat foods that contain energy such as protein, fats and carbohydrate, and also fruit and vegetables.
An increased appetite	1 Try to eat a balanced and sensible diet. 2 Plan your shopping to avoid impulse buys particularly of carbohydrates such as biscuits or chocolate. 3 In particular, try to avoid any increases in alcohol intake. It may add to your depression. 4 Try to eat meals while sitting at a meal table. Avoid snacking or bringing extra food to the table. If you want to eat more, force yourself to get up so that it is a conscious decision to eat it.
Increased weight	Reduced activity levels and increased appetite may cause weight gain. Think about: 1 Introducing some mild exercise into your day (this may also boost your mood).

Physical symptoms of depression	Hints and tips
Increased weight *(continued)*	2 Eating a balanced diet: vegetables and fruit will also prevent constipation.
Decreased weight	1 Eating a balanced range of foods is important to keep both your physical and mental strength up. 2 Try to keep eating a balanced range of foods that contain energy such as protein, fats and carbohydrate, and also fruit and vegetables.
Reduced energy	1 Low energy is a common problem in depression. 2 A vicious circle can arise. By reducing your activity, your muscles are used less. This causes them to weaken and feel painful and tired when they are used. 3 An effective way of overcoming this is to plan a **graded increase in your activity** in a step-by-step way. 4 This often leads to a **boost** in how you feel mentally as well as physically. 5 Remember, don't overdo exercise. Plan a **slow** increase in what you do. Just five minutes of exercise (e.g. walking up and downstairs three times a day to begin with) is the sort of level to aim at if you have not been doing any recent exercise. Slowly increase it over the next few days and weeks. 6 **If you have a physical illness**, please discuss this with your doctor and agree a plan for this graded increase in activity. 7 A common symptom in depression is to feel worse first thing in the morning. If you notice this, plan to do activities (such as going out) later on in the day. 8 Finally, don't throw yourself into this too quickly. Do it **one step at a time**.
A reduced sex drive	1 A reduced sex drive is common in depression. If you have a partner, try to discuss this with them. 2 Your sex drive will improve (as with other symptoms) towards its previous levels as you recover from depression. 3 In men, antidepressants can sometimes cause problems with having erections or ejaculating. If this is a difficulty for you and you are taking antidepressants, discuss this with your doctor. 4 If you find it difficult talking about this with a partner please do try to discuss it with your health care practitioner if this is a problem.

Symptoms of constipation	Constipation commonly occurs in depression.
	1 Simple changes can help:
	    ● eat vegetables, bran and fibre;
	    ● exercise helps constipation;
	    ● drink a reasonable amount of fluids.
	2 Constipation can be a side effect of some antidepressants.

Symptoms of pain	1 Pain such as chest pain, stomach pain and headaches may be worsened by depression. If this is the case, treating the depression is the best treatment. 2 If the pain is linked to the depression, you may find that painkillers such as aspirin and paracetamol do not seem to be very effective.

Physical symptoms of depression		Hints and tips
Symptoms of pain (continued)	3	If this is the case, it is important to avoid building up the dose of painkillers you are taking. This may cause new physical symptoms, and for some, painkillers may even cause more symptoms of pain and possibly addiction.
	4	In this case, treatment with antidepressants is often more effective. Please discuss this with your doctor.
Symptoms of physical agitation	1	Focusing your attention on them can sometimes worsen physical symptoms of agitation. This mental tension then adds to the unpleasant physical tension feelings.
	2	If the agitation feelings are very distressing, consider using medication to reduce it. Many effective short-term medications (which are not addictive) are available. In addition, antidepressant medication will often improve symptoms of agitation caused by depression. Discuss this with your doctor.

Workbook summary

In this workbook you have learned about:
- what are sleep and insomnia;
- common causes of sleep problems and actions you can take to help overcome problems of poor sleep;
- hints and tips for overcoming common physical problems that occur as part of depression.

Putting into practice what you have learned

Try to put into practice what you have learned during the next week. If you have difficulties with this workbook, don't worry. Just do what you can. If you have found any aspects of this workbook unhelpful, upsetting or confusing, please can you discuss this with your doctor or health care practitioner.

My notes

....

....

....

....

....

....

....

....

....

....

....

....

....

....

....

....

....

....

....

....

....

....

....

My notes

....

Workbook 9

Understanding and using antidepressant medication

Dr Chris Williams

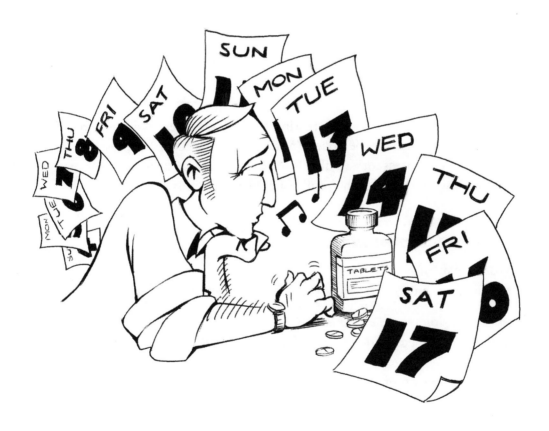

Overcoming Depression
A Five Areas Approach

Section 1 Introduction

This workbook is designed for anyone who is either taking antidepressant medication or who wishes to find out more about the uses of antidepressant medication.

In this workbook you will learn:
- why antidepressants may be used as a treatment for depression;
- about the advantages and disadvantages of taking antidepressant medication;
- about your own attitudes towards the use of antidepressants;
- ways of using antidepressants more effectively (if you are taking these).

Using antidepressants in the treatment of depression

If you are taking antidepressants:

Q. How long have you taken them for?	...... Years	...... Months
Q. Have they helped improve how you feel?	Yes ☐	No ☐
Q. Do you ever try to cope without them?	Yes ☐	No ☐
Q. Do you notice any side effects?	Yes ☐	No ☐

Antidepressants can be an important part of treating all aspects of depression. Because there are links between the altered thinking, feelings, behaviour and physical aspects of depression, the physical treatment offered by an antidepressant can also lead to positive improvements in negative, unhelpful and extreme thinking, low mood and unhelpfully altered behaviour.

The benefits of antidepressants

Who do they work best for?

A large number of different antidepressants exist. They are most often helpful when there is:

- significant depression *(low mood and a lack of enjoyment)*;
- several of the physical changes of depression *(low energy, reduced concentration, altered sleep or appetite)*;
- significant agitation or the onset or worsening of suspiciousness or panic;
- suicidal ideas: where you can't see a future.

How long do they take to work?

Normally, antidepressants take about **two weeks to begin to work** and their positive actions may take up to four to six weeks to reach a peak. It is very important therefore to take the tablets regularly and for long enough, even if to begin with they might seem like they are not working. Overall, around two thirds of patients respond to the first antidepressant medication they are prescribed. If there is little or no improvement, often an increase in dose or a change of medication will effectively treat the depression.

Warning: A common problem is that the person stops the antidepressants when they first feel well again. Stopping an antidepressant too early is a common cause of worsening depression. It is usually necessary to take the antidepressant medication for at least six months after feeling better to prevent slipping back into depression.

Do antidepressants have side effects?

All tablets have side effects. The important question is whether the side effects of having untreated depression are worse. Modern antidepressants are often **not** very sedating and do not cause very great weight gain. Many side effects disappear within a few days of starting the tablets as the body gets used to them. **Antidepressants are not addictive** however, if a person has taken the tablets for some time it is sensible for the dose of the antidepressant to be reduced slowly over a number of days before being stopped.

Antidepressants are the fastest and most effective way of improving depression in the short term if there is a significant physical aspect to your depression. If you are feeling very depressed, they can help you get to a stage where you are then able to look at making changes in your life to help prevent the depression occurring again. If you are taking an antidepressant, or wish to discuss whether taking one is likely to be helpful for you, you should discuss how your depression is best treated and whether you should take an antidepressant with your doctor. **Please do not stop taking antidepressants without the agreement of your doctor.**

Remembering to take antidepressants

For almost any medication, it may be difficult to remember to take them on a regular basis. This is particularly the case in depression because of the poor concentration and forgetfulness that can often occur.

Q. Do you sometimes forget to take your medication? Yes ☐ No ☐

Helpful hints:

The following may help you to remember to take your tablets:

1 Get into a **routine**: take the tablets at a set time each day.

2 **Place the tablets somewhere where you will see them** when you get up or go to bed (e.g. by your toothbrush). Avoid doing this if they may be taken by young children.

3 Write **little notes** to yourself saying *Medication* (or any other word to help remind you if you don't want others to read them). Stick them on the fridge, oven and back door so that you are reminded throughout the day).

Q. Do you ever get confused as to whether you have taken the medication? Yes ☐ No ☐

Helpful hints:

The following may help you be clear when you have taken your medication:

1 Tick off the doses you have taken in a **diary** or calendar.

2 If you are taking lots of tablets at different times each day, a **dosette box** can help. These have different compartments for each time of day so that you, or a friend, neighbour or health care practitioner can fill the box up in advance for the whole week. Ask your health care practitioner or pharmacist how to get one.

Q. Do you ever take a higher dose than is prescribed? Yes ☐ No ☐

KEY POINT

It is very important **not** to take a higher dose of antidepressant than your doctor prescribes. Antidepressant tablets work over a number of weeks. Taking more on one particular day will have **no** impact on your depression. It is the longer term taking them day in and day out at the correct dose that will lead to improvement. Tablets taken at higher than recommended doses may cause unpleasant side effects, or **potentially are dangerous**. Please do not do this. If you are concerned that an antidepressant is not working (remember they take at least two weeks to begin to work), please discuss this with your doctor.

My attitudes towards antidepressants

Antidepressant medications are sometimes viewed with suspicion. The following questions address some commonly held fears about antidepressant medication. Do you have any of these concerns?

Antidepressants are addictive   Yes ☐   No ☐

Useful information: It is not possible to become addicted to modern antidepressants in the same way as alcohol or tablets like diazepam. Antidepressants do need to be taken sensibly and as recommended by your doctor. If tablets are started at too high an initial dose, side effects are more common; similarly if a tablet taken at a high dose is stopped suddenly, some short-lived discontinuation symptoms may occur. To prevent this, many tablets are first started by slowly increasing the dose, and then later stopped by tapering down their dose over several days.

I should get better on my own without taking tablets   Yes ☐   No ☐

Antidepressants are often one of a number of ways of getting better. They work by treating some of the physical changes that occur in depression. They do not replace the need for you to identify and work at changing extreme or unhelpful thoughts and behaviours or the different practical problems you face. They can however be a useful additional way of improving how you feel. Your body, thoughts, and emotional feelings are all part of you – they are not in separate boxes. If you had broken a leg, you are unlikely to say *'I want to get better by myself without medical treatment'*. Why do the same in depression? If your doctor is recommending antidepressants, talk to him or her and discuss why they suggest this so that you can jointly make the decision about whether it is the right thing for you at the moment.

They cause side effects   Yes ☐   No ☐

All tablets cause side effects. The question is whether the **benefits** of taking the tablets outweigh the **costs**. Often side effects improve over the first few days of taking an antidepressant. Sometimes the dose of antidepressant can be reduced, or a different antidepressant with a different range of side effects can be prescribed. Please discuss this with your doctor.

On balance, have the antidepressants helped or hindered me?

If your answer to this is that they have helped, keep taking them as advised by your doctor. If you feel they have not helped you, please do not stop them yourself. Instead go and discuss this with your doctor. Perhaps the dose of the medication can be altered, or another medication may be more suitable. Whatever your decision, please do not decide to stop your medication without discussing it with your doctor.

- Antidepressants may have an important role in helping people with depression get better.

- Antidepressants are not addictive, however in stopping higher doses, it is sensible to slowly reduce the dose over a period of time.

- Taking the tablets on a regular basis is essential for them to work.

- All tablets have side effects; however for most people the benefits of antidepressants far outweigh the costs.

Summary

In this workbook you have learned about:

● why antidepressants may be used as a treatment for depression;
● the advantages and disadvantages of taking antidepressant medication;
● your own attitudes towards the use of antidepressants;
● ways of using antidepressants more effectively (if you are taking these).

Putting into practice what you have learned

Think about what you have learned during the next week. If you want to find out more about the use of antidepressants, or if you are having difficulties with your antidepressants (for example you are troubled by side effects, or they just don't seem to be working) please discuss this with your doctor or health care practitioner. If you have found any aspects of this workbook unhelpful, upsetting or confusing, please can you discuss this with your doctor or health care practitioner.

My notes

....

....

....

....

....

....

....

....

....

....

....

....

....

....

....

....

....

....

....

....

....

....

....

....

My notes

....

Workbook 10
Planning for the future

Dr Chris Williams

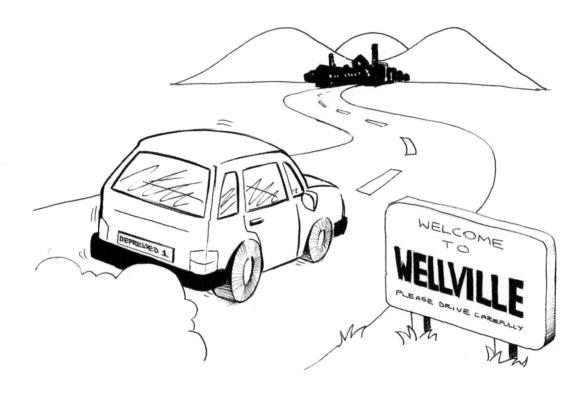

Overcoming Depression
A Five Areas Approach

Section 1   **Introduction**

In this workbook you will:

- summarise what you have learned about getting better and create a plan to use if you begin to feel worse again in future;
- produce a list of your own 'early warning signs' to help you watch out for signs of worsening depression;
- find out about how to set up your own regular review session to help you put into practice what you have learned.

Planning for the future

This section summarises some principles that you may find helpful when it comes to planning how to face the future. It can sometimes be helpful to think of yourself as being on a journey of recovery. When you first started working on your problems, it is likely that you had a range of different problems you wished to tackle. During the treatment, it is to be hoped, things have improved in at least some areas since you began your journey down this path.

The following are some questions to help you identify **what** has been helpful for you and what things have helped you move on. Write down your thoughts in the space below each question:

My journey:

Q. What is different now from before? What gains have I made? How have I improved in each of the five areas of depression?

- In my thinking?

✎

- In my feelings?

✎

- In my behaviour?

✎

- In the practical situations, relationships and practical problems that I face?

✎

Q. What have I done to make this happen?

● In my thinking?

✎

● In my actions?

✎

Q. How can I apply these changes to future problems?

✎

Q. What new skills have I gained that I can use to help me continue to improve?

✎

Q. How can I continue to use what I have learned in my everyday life?

✎

Q. What things might get in the way of me doing this? How can I deal with these obstacles? What practical steps can I take?

Try to see if you can summarise what you have learned as **general rules** that you can apply in life. You can write as many or as few rules as you want. The following example summarises what Paul (who had experienced problems of depression) has learned:

Example – Paul's rules for life:

1 *When I begin to feel depressed, I need to do something about it before it worsens.*
2 *I **can** control my negative thoughts by using the thought worksheets.*
3 *Don't withdraw from others when I feel down – they can really help me pick up.*
4 *Avoid drinking too much – it only makes things worse.*
5 *When I feel overwhelmed by problems – just tackle them one at a time.*

Now, try this for yourself

Q. What have you learned about getting and staying better?

✎ My rules for life

1

2

3

4

5

Looking for signs of relapse

One of the most important things is to be aware of vulnerable times so that you can plan out in advance what to do if you are beginning to feel worse for whatever reason. Sometimes, certain situations make people feel especially bad or seem particularly difficult to cope with. Everyone is different. Different problems may affect people in very different ways. They could include times such as:

● when you feel let down, rejected or abandoned by someone (e.g. after a relationship difficulty or breakdown);
● after something important seems to have either gone wrong or you have a fear that it will go wrong;
● when you think things are beginning to get out of control.

Q. What are *my* possible *high-risk situations* in terms of setbacks?

1

2

3

Q. What do I need to do differently if I encounter these situations?

1

2

3

Watch for early warning signs

One helpful approach is to try to watch out for early signs that problems such as depression or anxiety are returning. Try to write out a short list of warning signs to watch out for. This may include things like:

- *Altered thinking*

  Noticing increased extreme, negative or unhelpful thoughts that begin to dominate your mind.

- *Altered feelings*

  Such as feeling down and low.

- *Altered behaviour – reduced activities*

  Beginning to withdraw from others or activities (**reduced activity**) or to increasingly avoid certain situations (e.g. by staying in bed later and later).

- *Altered behaviour – unhelpful activities*

  Drinking more alcohol or carrying out other **unhelpful activities** as a means of blocking how you feel.

- *Altered physical symptoms*

  For example, of growing tension or restlessness, or a worsening of your sleep or appetite.

- *Situation, relationship and practical problems*

  A build-up of problems that begin to feel overwhelming.

The following example summarises how Muriel looked back to identify her own early warning signs of recurring depression.

Example: Muriel's early warning signs

Muriel has identified that her early warning signs are:

- *Altered thinking*   Becoming very negative and predicting that things will go badly (negative predictions). Having a very negative view of myself. Overlooking good things that happen (mental filter).

- *Altered feelings*   Feeling low and weepy, and also feeling very little at all, as though my emotions are becoming numb.

- *Altered behaviour*   A tendency to want to withdraw and ask my sister not to visit. Stopping doing things I normally enjoy such as going for a walk or going to the shops.

- *Altered physical feelings/symptoms*   Feeling very low in energy and finding it difficult getting up in the morning.

- *Situation, relationship and practical problems*   Feeling overwhelmed by problems and not acting to overcome them.

In addition, it can be helpful if Muriel can identify one ***key early warning sign***. This should be a key symptom that she can watch for and that was present quite early on when she became depressed before.

My key early warning sign:

'I am going to watch out for times when I feel really tired, not just a bit tired, but times when I feel exhausted all the time and just want to stay in bed.'

This key early warning sign means: **Do something now to treat the depression**.

Example: Paul's early warning signs

Paul has identified that his early warning signs are:

- *Altered thinking*   Mind-reading that others don't like me. Losing confidence. Predicting the worst will happen (catastrophising).

- *Altered feelings*   Feeling low and weepy.

- *Altered behaviour*   Trying to block how I feel by drinking more than normal. Beginning to avoid things that seem scary.

- *Altered physical symptoms*   Feeling really tense and jittery.

- *Situation, relationship and practical problems*   Beginning to put off handing work in, and becoming unassertive in sorting things out. Letting problems go unaddressed.

My key early warning sign:

'I am going to watch out for times when I feel I lose confidence and start mind-reading what others think of me.'

Now, try to create **your own** list of early warning signs:

My early warning signs

- ✎ *Altered thinking:*

- ✎ *Altered feelings:*

- ✎ *Altered behaviour:*

- ✎ *Altered physical symptoms:*

- *Situation, relationship and practical problems:*

My key early warning sign:

If you notice this **key early warning sign**, this means **do something <u>now</u> about the depression**.

Sometimes it can help to also talk to others who you know and trust to discover if they have noticed any other early warning signs. If they notice any, you could watch for these yourself, and also ask them to tell you if they notice these themselves.

The purpose of creating this early warning list is so that you can plan how to deal with any future worsening of how you feel at an early stage.

What do you need to do if you start to experience these early warning signs in order to reduce the chances of them leading on to worsening symptoms?

Producing an emergency plan

Imagine you live in a house, which has a smoke detector. One day you hear it beeping while you are watching television. What do you do – do you ignore it and keep watching the television as if there was no problem – or do you get up, find out if there is a problem and try to deal with it? In the same way, if you notice any of your *early warning signs*, you need to have planned what you do in response.

This might include things such as planning to make changes:

In your thinking:

- Stop, think and reflect on your thoughts.

- Go and talk to a health care practitioner about your problems and discuss if you need any other help such as an antidepressant or to see a mental health specialist such as a clinical psychologist, psychiatrist or a nurse.

- **If you have used them,** to use the thought investigation and challenge worksheets workbooks 4 and 5 to identify and change unhelpful and extreme thinking.

In your behaviour:

- Choose to stay in contact with people who may support you. Choose not to isolate yourself – tell others you trust that you are noticing some problems.

- Tackle avoidance of people or places by going into places you may have recently begun to avoid.

- **If you have used this approach,** create an action plan to plan your activities – use workbook 6 to help you do this.

An **emergency plan** can help you to plan out how to tackle any early warning signs you notice. The following example shows how Muriel decides to react to her early warning signs.

Example: Muriel's emergency plan

Early warning sign	Emergency plan
Altered thinking: with negative predictions and mind-reading.	To identify and challenge extreme and unhelpful thinking.
Altered behaviour: withdrawing from doing things I like.	Create an **action plan** to do things that give me a sense of pleasure and achievement.
Altered behaviour: asking my sister Mary not to visit.	Choose to ask Mary over each week for a short period of time.
Altered physical symptoms: feeling low in energy, and worse in the morning.	Plan to do more difficult tasks later on in the day. Do things at a reasonable pace.
Altered feelings: Feeling low and weepy.	Do all the above things, and also go to see my doctor to talk about whether other treatments such as an antidepressant may be useful.

My emergency plan

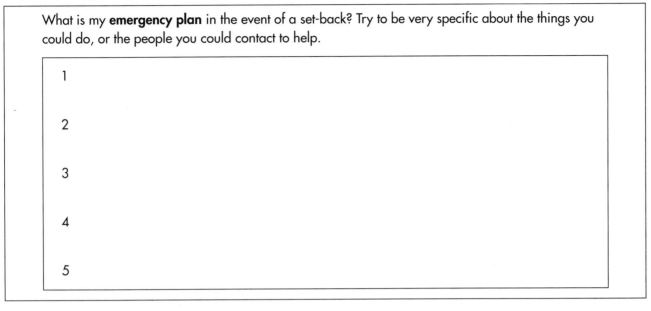

What is my **emergency plan** in the event of a set-back? Try to be very specific about the things you could do, or the people you could contact to help.

1

2

3

4

5

If the problems begin to worsen in spite of your plan, go to the professionals. If a fire was beginning to worsen at home in spite of your attempts to tackle it, you would call for professional help. Similarly, if you feel worse in spite of your emergency plan, get in touch with your previous health care practitioner or your doctor. They will be able to help advise you as to whether other additional approaches such as the use of medication may be helpful.

The concept of a regular review session

It is important to **continue** using the information and skills that you have learned during the next few months and into the future. One of the advantages of using a workbook such as this one is that it allows you to set particular goals, and review how things have gone. You can also **do this yourself** by setting up a **regular review session**.

How to develop a regular review session

- Get a pen and mark the last day of each month as a '**review session**' on your calendar.
- During this **review session**, try to spend 30 minutes or so to think back over the previous month.

Review session: How has the month gone?

Q. Try to think about things that have gone well and allow yourself to experience pleasure when thinking about this.

● What things have gone well?

✎ Write them down here:

Q. If some areas haven't gone as well as you would have liked, write them down here:

✎

Q. Try to work out what it was about the difficult situation that led this to happen?

✎

Q. Was there anything you could have done differently?

✎

Q. How could you deal with it differently in future?

✎

Write an **action plan** that you can put into practice over the following month. Try to set specific goals and targets. Plan in some activities that will lead you to have a sense of achievement or pleasure or to overcome problems such as avoidance or other unhelpful activities.

● Plan things in a step-by-step way, being very specific about what you want to do and trying to be realistic in what it is possible to achieve.

● How will you try to make sure that you carry out your plan?

● What can prevent this happening? What might sabotage your plan?

● How can you overcome any problems?

You can do this review session more often (e.g. every 2 weeks) if you find this helpful. The purpose is to spend a little time to stop, think and reflect, and plan how to move forwards.

Finally, remember that you are not alone. Your health care practitioner or doctor is there as a resource to work with you and help you move forwards. You can discuss any problems or difficulties with them.

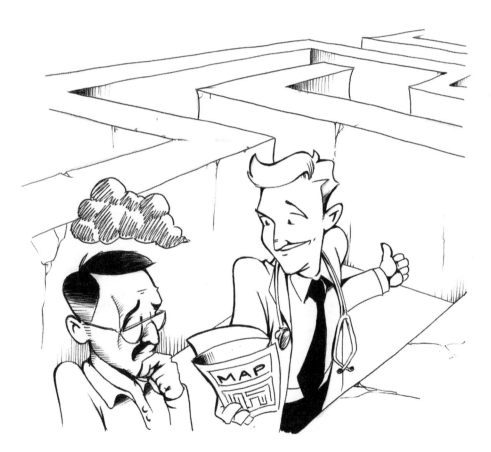

Workbook summary

In this workbook you have learned about:

- summarising what you have learned about getting better and creating a plan to use if you begin to feel worse again in future;
- producing a list of your own 'early warning signs' to help you watch out for signs of worsening depression;
- how to set up your own regular review session to help you put into practice what you have learned.

Putting into practice what you have learned

You may find it helpful to re-read this and other workbooks on a regular basis. Consider building this reading into your regular review sessions.

If you have found any aspects of this workbook unhelpful, upsetting or confusing, please can you discuss this with your doctor or health care practitioner.

My notes

....

....

....

....

....

....

....

....

....

....

....

....

....

....

....

....

....

....

....

....

....

....

....

....

....

My notes

....

Part 2

The assessment and management of depression

Section 1 Notes for health care practitioners

How often should a progress review occur?

The workbooks have been devised to be used at home by the person with depression in conjunction with short review or monitoring sessions with their health care practitioner. This might typically occur once a fortnight or so. At shortest, a seven to eight minute review will allow a discussion of areas that are going well, areas that they are having problems with, and will allow the person to be given the next workbook to work on at home. Workers from some professional groups may have more time available for the review sessions. In cases where additional time is available, specific components of the course can be discussed or looked at in more detail (for example a completed thought challenge worksheet could be discussed).

In short, the balance and length of sessions can be jointly agreed with the person based on the realities of available time, and individual preference.

The workbooks '*do the work*' of providing an effective psychosocial intervention by:
- providing important information.
- asking sequences of questions in a way that helps the reader begin to understand their symptoms (unhelpful thoughts and behaviours) and start to change them in a step by step way.

Working to overcome common difficulties in using the workbooks

Self-help approaches can be a helpful and acceptable form of treatment for many. Of those offered this approach, some will initially start using the workbooks, and then run into difficulties. The following summarises some common problems encountered, and suggests practical ways that you can helpfully work jointly to overcome these difficulties.

I didn't have time to do it

Breaking old habits and starting new ones takes practice. They have the **right** to set aside time to change. Getting better should be a priority. It may be that they think that they have too many external pressures (e.g. a partner, children or job) to look after their own needs. It is, however, important for the person and for those around them that they spend time to allow themselves to get better.

I didn't understand what I had to do

If the reader feels stuck, encourage them to try to re-read the workbook again. If they are still confused, encourage them to talk to you about any particular difficulties they may have with understanding what to do.

I tried but it didn't seem to make any difference

Change takes time. The person may have been depressed for quite some time and it will take time to begin to change. The first steps to change are often the most difficult. Try to encourage them to stick at it. Learning to overcome depression involves learning new *knowledge* about the causes of depression, and gaining new *skills* in overcoming it. Although it can take time to learn these, they **can** change one step at a time.

Intervention

Sometimes it is easy to forget how difficult it is to learn new information or skills that we now take for granted. Ask them to think about some of the skills they have learned over the years. For example, if they can drive, ask them to think back to their **first driving lesson**. It is unlikely they were very good at driving that first time, yet with practice they developed the new knowledge and skills needed to drive. They can learn skills in overcoming depression in the same way. It may seem difficult at first but they need to keep practising what they learn. If they don't drive, encourage them to think of other things they can now do that originally took time to grasp. They may have been difficult at the time, but they managed in the end.

If the person is moderately depressed and is experiencing many physical (biological) symptoms of depression, consider whether to suggest prescribing an antidepressant in addition to using the workbooks (see **section 2**).

Try to help them challenge any negative thoughts about the possibility of improvement by asking: 'What advice would you give to a friend who said "*I'll never change?*"' Often people can give far better advice to someone else than they give to themselves. Use this to illustrate this '*one rule for you, another for others*' and ask them to follow their own good advice – 'If you would offer this advice to a friend, then why not also offer it to yourself?'

Completing the tasks set out in each workbook is an important part of changing. It is the day-to-day practice of these tasks that will help them get better.

In addition, a further short handout has been prepared which can be provided if motivation is a problem. This can be worked though at home and then discussed at the next appointment. The handout '*Overcoming low motivation*' is included as appendix 1 at the end. A second handout addressing the common question '*What is the cause of my depression?*' is included as appendix 2.

A note for non-mental health specialists:
Referral should occur to the local psychiatric team for risk assessment and management in any cases where suicidal ideas or significant hopelessness are present or suspected.

Additional resources

Additional workbooks and other resources (for example details of group treatment resources) are available through our web-site www.calipso.co.uk

Copyright

The materials are copyright of Dr Chris Williams and the University of Leeds Innovations Ltd 2001.

- A photocopying licence has been granted to allow purchasers of the *Overcoming Depression* book to make **multiple copies** of the workbooks for use clinically or in teaching.

Overcoming Depression **training events**

You may find that completing the workbooks yourself helps you obtain a firm grasp of the content and purpose of each workbook. A range of training events are also available to familiarise you with the materials and how to use them effectively.

● An accompanying training CD Rom illustrates the use of the five areas approach with Muriel and Paul from the *Overcoming Depression* course.

● Training courses from half day to four days, are offered to interested groups. Please find out more at our web-site **www.Calipso.co.uk** or via Dr Chris Williams **chrisw@fiveareas.com**

Contact details for copies of the training CD Rom and other training materials:

Stephen Taylor-Parker,
University of Leeds Innovations Ltd,
175 Woodhouse Lane, Leeds LS2 3AR.
Tel. 0113 233 3444   Fax. 0113 234 3811   E-mail. s.taylor-parker@ulis.co.uk

---

Section 2 Detecting and treating depression: a guide for non-mental health professionals

Detection of depression is important as treatment shortens the duration of the episode and results in less long-term social impairment.

How to detect depression

- **Consider** depression as a possibility.

- Pay attention to verbal and non-verbal cues.

- Make early eye contact.

- Clarify the presenting complaint.

- Ask 'open' questions and later use more specific 'closed' questions.

- Spend less time talking and interrupt less.

- Seem less rushed.

- Show empathy.

- Ask about family, work and social issues.

Consider depression if:

- there is a clear change from their normal self.

- general physical complaints are made ('tired', 'can't sleep', 'washed out', 'stressed') or increased consultation/requests for tests occur.

- objectively inappropriate requests for urgent attention are seen.

- tears or angry outbursts occur during the consultation.

- excessive anxiety about family members or about their own health (hypochondriasis or somatisation) is seen.

- weight loss, reduced appetite or insomnia are the presenting complaints.

- the person says they are no longer coping.

Questions based on Craig and Boardman (1997).

Key symptoms of a depressive disorder/illness:

● altered thinking (e.g. negative, extreme thoughts, themes of being guilty, hopeless, and/or suicidal ideas);

● altered mood (low mood/loss of pleasure for two or more weeks);

● altered physical changes (sleep, energy, appetite, weight, concentration, diurnal variation – worse first thing in the morning);

● altered behaviour (impact on social functioning/reduced activity, unhelpful behaviours).

Poor outcome is associated with:

● delayed or insufficient initial treatment;

● continuing problems in family, marriage or employment;

● more severe illness;

● co-morbid physical illness.

(Craig and Boardman, 1997).

Antidepressants are effective treatments for depressive disorder. They tend to be more effective in moderate and severe depressive disorders than in mild depression.

If antidepressants are appropriate and prescribed, remember to offer:

● an adequate dose (easier when Selective Serotonin Re-uptake Inhibitors – SSRIs – are used, as the starting dose is also often an effective therapeutic dose);
● adequate time – allow four to six weeks or more at an effective dose before a change of medication for non-response should be considered;
● careful monitoring and education about the need for ongoing medication (if prescribed);
● remember, most people prescribed antidepressants stop them within three weeks as a result of poor compliance.

The *Overcoming Depression* course is not intended to train you as an expert in cognitive behaviour therapy. If the person requires specialist psychiatric or psychological therapy input, referral should be made in the normal way for specialist assessment.

Reference

Craig, T.K.J. and Boardman, A.P. (1997) Common mental health problems in primary care. *British Medical Journal*, 314, 1609–12.

Appendix 1   **Overcoming low motivation**

It can sometimes be difficult trying to change when you feel depressed. Many things can interfere or get in the way of working on overcoming your problems. Listed below are some of them.

I didn't have the time to do it
Breaking old habits and starting new ones takes practice. You have the **right** to set aside time to change. Getting better should be a priority. It may be that you think that you have too many external pressures (e.g. a partner, children or job) to look after your own needs. It is, however, important for you and for those around you that you spend time to allow yourself to get better.

I didn't understand what I had to do
If you feel stuck, try to re-read the workbook again. If you are still confused, talk to the health care practitioner who introduced you to the course about any difficulties you may have with understanding what to do.

I tried but it didn't seem to make any difference
Change takes time. You may have been depressed for quite some time now and it will take time to begin to change. The first steps to change are often the most difficult. Try to encourage yourself to stick at it.

I don't think it will help me get better
One of the biggest blocks to getting better is not believing you can change. If you believe that change is not possible and decide to do nothing as a result, you may end up missing out on real benefits. Change is possible. Making negative predictions that nothing will happen may become a self-fulfilling prophecy that will **prevent** you getting better.

Try to challenge any negative thoughts about the possibility of improvement by asking yourself the following questions:

Q. Is change possible for me?

Learning to overcome depression involves learning new *knowledge* about the causes of depression, and learning new *skills* in overcoming it. Although it can take time to learn these, you **can** change one step at a time.

Sometimes it is easy to forget how difficult it is to learn new information or skills that you now take for granted. Think about some of the skills you have learned over the years. For example, if you can drive, think back to your first driving lesson. It is unlikely you were very good at driving that first time, yet with practice you developed the new knowledge and skills needed to drive. You can overcome depression in the same way. It may seem difficult at first but keep practising what you learn. If you don't drive, think of other things you can now do which took time to learn. They may have been difficult at the time, but you managed.

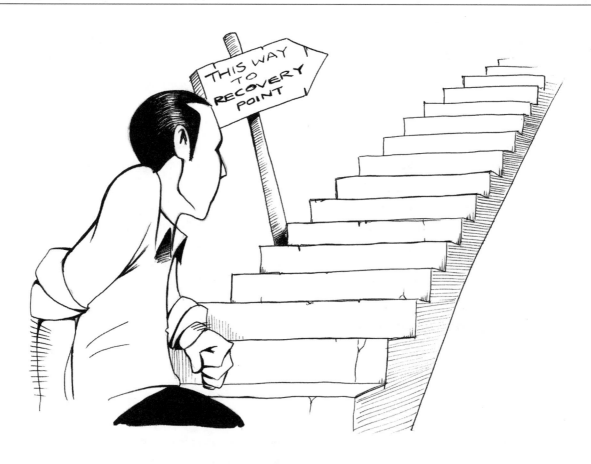

✎ Write down what other things you have learnt that took time:

Identifying any blocking thoughts

Sometimes thinking negatively can undermine confidence and stop people believing they can change. What you think can affect both how you **feel** and what you **do**. Often when someone thinks negatively and jumps to conclusions, what they believe **is not actually true**. If they **stop to think and reflect,** they can often find many reasons why their negative thoughts are inaccurate. One way of describing this is that most extreme beliefs are both unhelpful and untrue.

Challenging blocking thoughts

For example, trying to distance yourself from your negative blocking thoughts can help you be more objective. What advice would you give to a friend who said '*I'll never change*'? Would you say:

Q. Okay, that's fine. You don't need to.		Yes ☐	No ☐
Q. Keep trying. Don't give up. You can change bit by bit.		Yes ☐	No ☐
Q. Forget it, you're useless. Don't bother, you'll never change.		Yes ☐	No ☐

If a friend told you '*I'll never change*' it would be most helpful for you to encourage them. They need encouragement particularly at times they believe nothing can change.

✎ What would you say to them? Write it down here:

If you would offer this advice to a friend, then why not also offer it to yourself?

Completing the tasks set out in each workbook is an important part of changing. It is the day-to-day practice of these tasks that will help you get you better. This will help you to bring the workbooks into your everyday week to help you to *stop, think and reflect* on how you are feeling. You may believe at first that nothing is changing, but slowly you will notice positive change.

Appendix 2   **What are the causes of my depression?**

Why do people develop depression?

The following areas are known to play a part in the causes of depression. Not every factor is present in every case.

- Situation, relationship and practical problems
- Psychological factors
- Physical factors

Situation, relationship and practical problems contributing to depression

When someone faces a large number of problems they may begin to feel overwhelmed and depressed. Dwelling on the problems may worsen things still further and quickly get them out of proportion. The problem is unhelpfully focused on and mulled over again and again in a way that doesn't help resolve it. This **unhelpful focus** can worsen how you feel. It can also be unhelpful because the result is that the person can feel unable to know where to start to change things.

These problems may include:

- debts, housing or other difficulties;

- problems in relationships with family, friends or colleagues, etc.;

- other difficult situations that you face.

Vulnerability to depression is often linked with **stresses** at home or work (or lack of work – for example **unemployment**). People who have suffered a relationship split, or who feel isolated with no one to talk to about how they feel are also prone to depression. Young mothers, and mothers facing the demands of trying to bring up many young children are also at greater risk of depression. At the same time, sometimes practical and helpful supports may be available through friends or relatives.

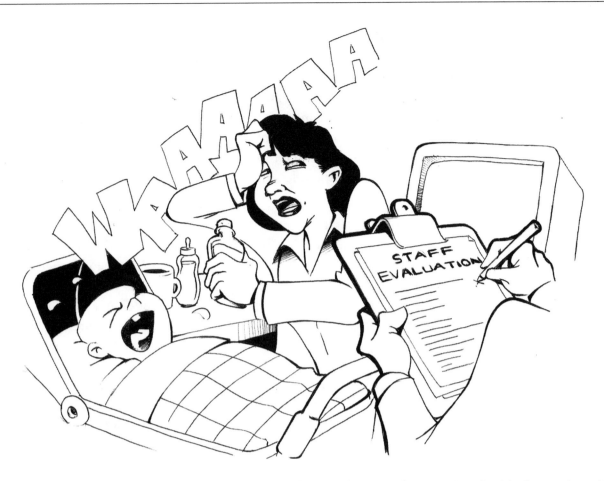

The following table summarises several common factors that may be associated with depression. Are any of these relevant to you?

Situation, relationship and practical problems

I have relationship difficulties (such as arguments) with: Yes ☐   No ☐

✎ *(write in the person's name or initials)*

I can't really talk and receive support from my partner.	Yes ☐	No ☐
There is no one around whom I can really talk to.	Yes ☐	No ☐
I feel stressed by the demands of looking after my children.	Yes ☐	No ☐
I have difficulties with money worries or debts.	Yes ☐	No ☐
I don't like where I live.	Yes ☐	No ☐
I am having problems with my neighbours.	Yes ☐	No ☐
I feel upset by my lack of a job.	Yes ☐	No ☐
I don't enjoy my job.	Yes ☐	No ☐
I have difficulties with colleagues at work.	Yes ☐	No ☐

Psychological factors contributing to depression

A number of psychological (thinking) factors are important in the cause of depression. Sometimes unhelpful extreme and negative thinking can be started or worsened by a **loss event** (e.g. the breakdown of a relationship, loss of a job), or the **threat of such a loss** occurring. Sometimes, depression occurs when the person feels overwhelmed by the problems they face. Psychological factors are very important in understanding these different reactions.

People are very different in how they respond to such loss events and to the different stresses that they face. One key factor is the importance of the **rules** that we all learn as we grow up.

Our inner rules

As we grow up, we each learn important rules about how we understand and make sense of ourselves and the people and events around us. It is in childhood that these central ways of seeing things are first learned. They may be affected by our relationship with important people such as our parent or parents, brothers or sisters and whether we have received love, consistency and support. Sometimes the opposite occurs – rejection and inconsistency, and this can undermine us as we grow up. These central ways of seeing things are sometimes called **core beliefs**. Common core beliefs may be based around positive themes such as seeing yourself as competent and successful, or more negative themes such as being a failure, bad, unlovable, incompetent, foolish or weak. Most people develop a range of both positive and negative core beliefs during their childhood.

Even if someone has a very happy upbringing, it is common for them to have at least some negative beliefs about how they see themselves or others. Even if someone is usually not troubled by more negative and unhelpful core beliefs, if depression becomes more severe, the few they have may still come to dominate their thinking and lead to a wide range of extreme and unhelpful ways of thinking and acting.

For most of our lives we may be only partially aware of these core beliefs, and if they are noticed, most people who are not depressed can quite quickly challenge and deal with any fleeting unhelpful core beliefs that come into mind.

Psychological factors such as extreme and unhelpful thinking are very much a part of depression and have their roots in unhelpful core beliefs. Psychological factors can sometimes also be important in understanding the **causes** of depression. For example, long-term low self-esteem is a risk factor for depression. In addition, when someone experiences either a **loss event** (for example a relationship ends or a close relative dies) or a **threatened loss** (e.g. the threat of unemployment or failure), this can lead to the core beliefs becoming more dominant. Extreme and unhelpful thoughts begin to intrude more and more into consciousness and lead to the range of altered thinking, emotions, behaviour and physical reactions.

The following table summarises several common factors that may be associated with depression. Are any of these relevant to you?

Psychological factors affecting my depression:		
I experienced a recent loss event in my life.	Yes ☐	No ☐
I am facing a threatened loss event in my life now.	Yes ☐	No ☐
I experienced many upsets at home when I grew up.	Yes ☐	No ☐
I experienced many upsets at school (such as being bullied) when I grew up.	Yes ☐	No ☐

Physical factors contributing to depression

Physical changes are a recognised part of a depressive illness. Physical factors, such as a deficiency of chemicals in the brain known as amines occurs in severe depression. Sometimes this occurs after a stress, such as a loss, or a large **life event**. These changes may also be caused by:

- certain drugs or medications that lower amine levels in the brain and can cause depression.
- physical illnesses (e.g. anaemia, lowered thyroid function, and heart disease) are amongst a range of physical illnesses that can cause depression. That is why it is important to have a proper physical examination and sometimes blood tests when you are depressed. If you have not had these, discuss whether they are needed with your doctor.
- excessive alcohol or the use of many illegal drugs may contribute to lowering mood.

What about genetics?

Studies show that in cases of very severe depression, there is an increased risk that other relatives have also experienced psychiatric disorders such as depression or problems with alcohol. Just because a close relative has experienced depression does not mean that this is the reason why **you** are depressed. It may be part of the reason, but in most cases other factors such as practical problems or psychological factors are also present.

The following table summarises several common factors that may be associated with depression. Are any of these relevant to you?

Physical factors affecting my depression:		
I haven't had a physical examination and blood tests.	Yes ☐	No ☐
I may be drinking too much.	Yes ☐	No ☐
I have a close relative who has experienced depression or alcohol problems.	Yes ☐	No ☐
I have a chronic illness/health problem.	Yes ☐	No ☐

You may wish to discuss these different areas with your health care practitioner.

Index